FINISH LINE FUELING

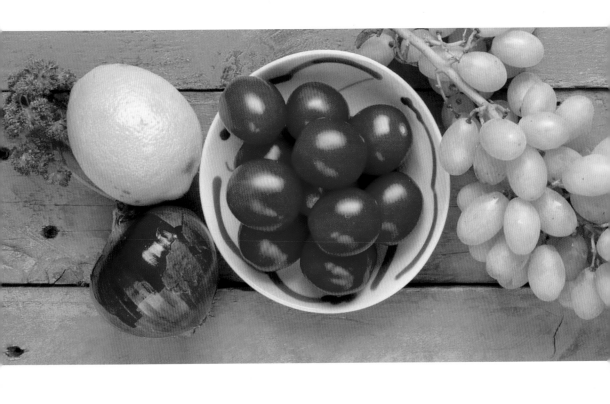

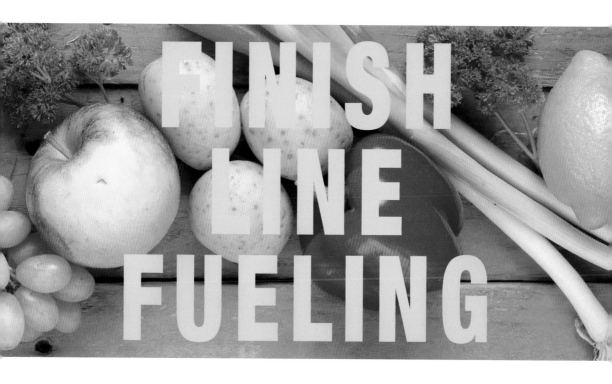

FINISH LINE FUELING

AN ESSENTIAL GUIDE TO RUNNER'S NUTRITION

JACKIE DIKOS, RD, CSSD, CLT

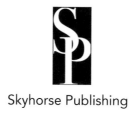

Skyhorse Publishing

Skyhorse Publishing books may be purchased in bulk at special discounts for sales promotion, corporate gifts, fund-raising, or educational purposes. Special editions can also be created to specifications. For details, contact the Special Sales Department, Skyhorse Publishing, 307 West 36th Street, 11th Floor, New York, NY 10018 or info@skyhorsepublishing.com.

Skyhorse® and Skyhorse Publishing® are registered trademarks of Skyhorse Publishing, Inc.®, a Delaware corporation.

Visit our website at www.skyhorsepublishing.com.

10 9 8 7 6 5 4 3 2 1

Library of Congress Cataloging-in-Publication Data is available on file.

Cover design by Tom Lau
Cover photo credit: iStockphoto
Interior photographs by Jonathon Fean and Jackie Dikos

Print ISBN: 978-1-5107-1962-0
Ebook ISBN: 978-1-5107-1964-4

Printed in China

Contents

For Greg and our race without a finish line.

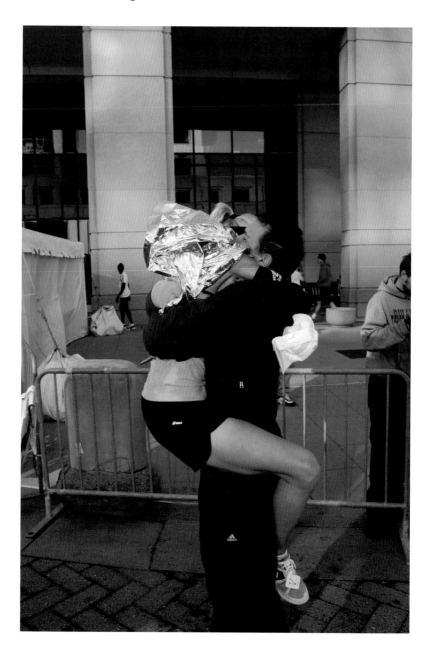

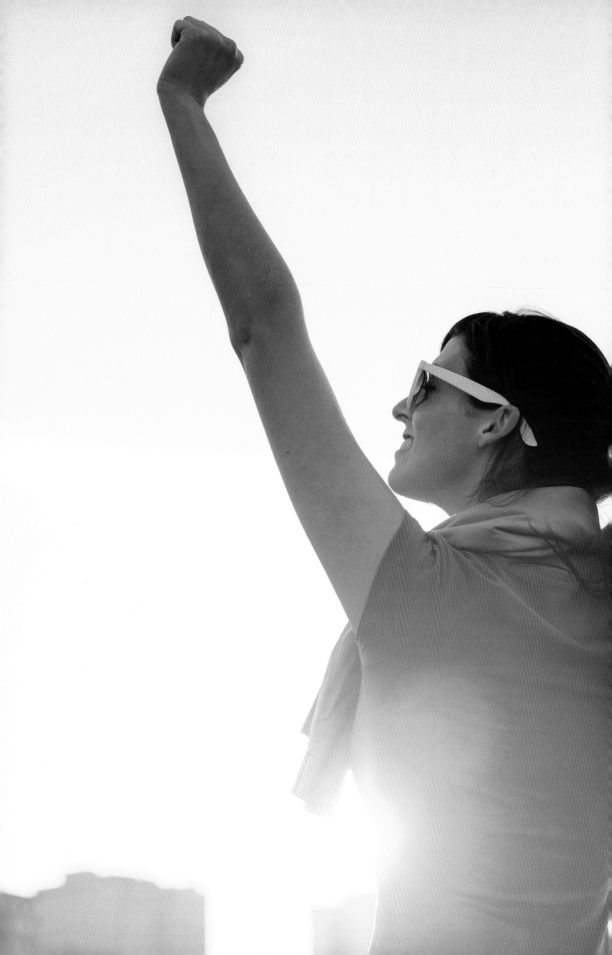

Introduction

Quality of Life: What Does It Mean to You?

Early in my career as a dietitian, I worked in the hospital setting. While there, I found that there were many circumstances when patients and doctors were making decisions based on what patients wanted most in regards to quality of life. Decisions ranged from a medication choice, whether to have an elective surgery to increase activity level, or to concede and stop treatments in order to be more comfortable at the end of life.

These decisions often slipped into my conversations at home with my husband when I was at my peak of training 80 to 100 miles a week. My husband, Greg, is an orthopedic trauma surgeon who faces quality of life decisions with patients daily. In the midst of heavy training, raising our young son, and working as a dietitian he would frequently remind me that I did not "have" to run. It was a choice I made in regards to what I wanted from life each day I squeezed in the demanding schedule.

As I prepared for the start of my first marathon as a runner of sub-elite status, Greg reminded me to take many mental "photos" of the special opportunity. I have many amazing mental images of that day. It was my first qualification for the Olympic Team Trials Marathon and the product of what I had pushed through each sluggish morning. It was a powerful reminder that I felt blessed with an amazing quality of life.

These experiences, and many like it, have offered me great perspective. The phrase "quality of life" has become my personal motto and the focus for those I educate. Every day, as athletes and as people, we face decisions. It may be what to eat or drink, or whether to run on a bitter cold morning. Each decision plays a role in how we interpret both short-term and long-term quality of life goals. How will each decision support what I want most from life and my future?

I find quality of life pieces come together when I avoid overcomplicating decisions—including training and food. There is more to everyday fueling than calories-in and calories-out in an effort to optimize nutritional status, health, and performance. My goal for the pages ahead is to help the runner better understand what the body requires on an individual level, interpret how the body communicates needs, and how to respond to support both quality of life and performance related goals.

My quality of life goals: to feel happy, healthy, and unstoppable.

Happy: Part of a world full of life, love, and potential. Slow to anger, quick to respond, and confident in my own skin.

Healthy: Free from pain, excessive fatigue, and chronic disease.

Unstoppable: A feeling of infinite energy and sense of limitless potential for the day. To be as productive as possible.

—Jackie Dikos, RD, CSSD, CLT

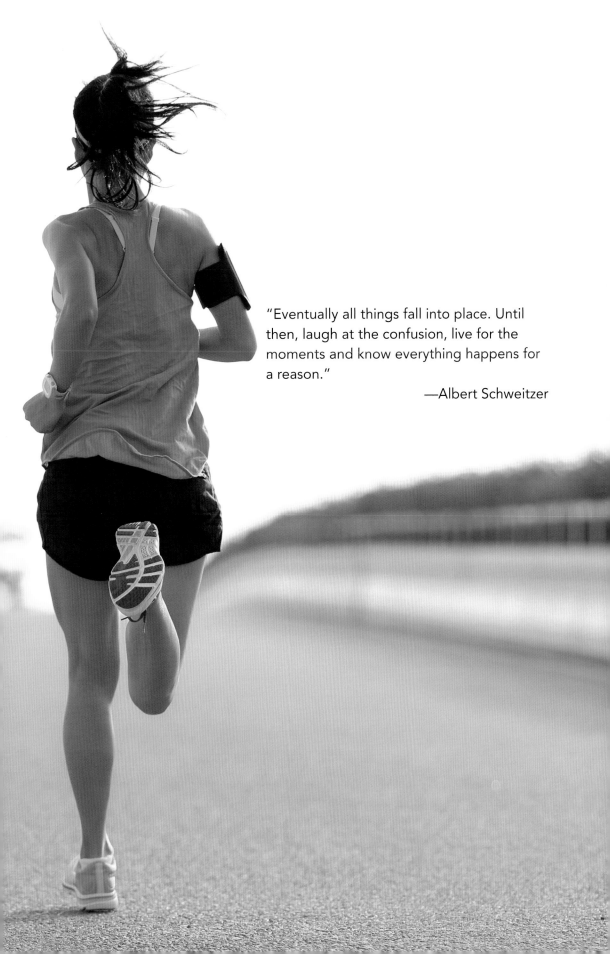

"Eventually all things fall into place. Until then, laugh at the confusion, live for the moments and know everything happens for a reason."

—Albert Schweitzer

GOAL-SETTING ESSENTIALS FOR EVERYDAY HEALTH AND OPTIMAL PERFORMANCE

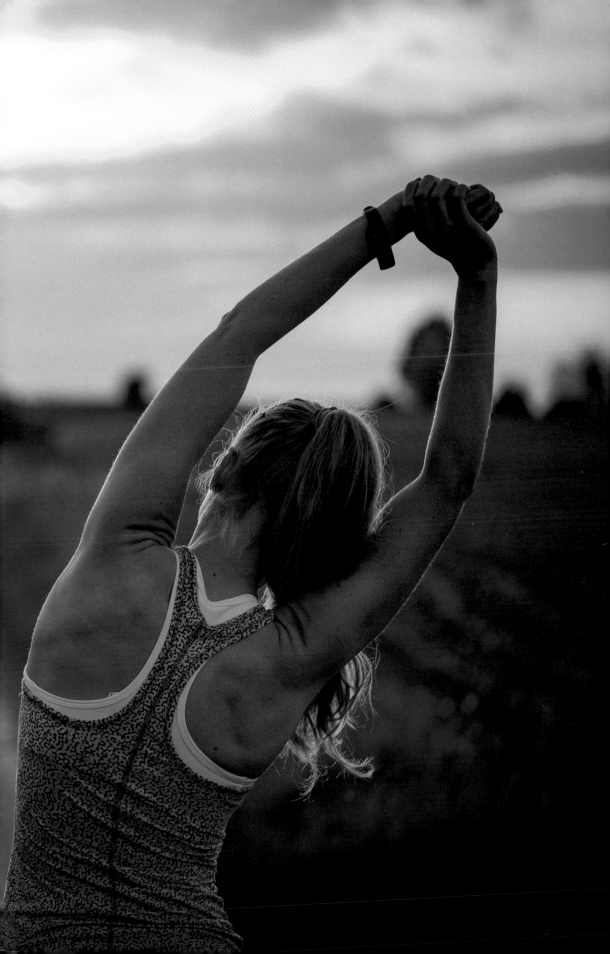

What does a loyal runner want most from his or her day? They want to run. A day without taking in the fresh air, working up good sweat, and feeling the smooth rhythm of a spirited stride feels like it's missing something. A run makes the day feel more complete.

Feeling great when we run—now that's a state of contentment beyond measure. It feels like cashing in a winning lottery ticket. It makes a good day brighten into a great one with an extra ray of sunshine. The lasting state of contentment that comes with a great run makes the countless miles and endless effort of basic daily training worth every tiresome second.

When we just want to run, everything else, including food, seems to just complicate things. One more mile on a run can easily take precedence over post-run flexibility and refueling. Long workouts, a busy schedule, and working in enough sleep to do it all over again can demand a lot out of the day. Over time the pantry becomes lined with prepackaged foods, sports performance energy products, and fad diet books in an effort to find simple answers to support efficiency in life and performance. The message of what entails quality fueling and goals to support performance can get muddled.

Food doesn't have to be complicated. Keeping food simple and making the effort to put together basic food choices can fuel even the most demanding lifestyle. Bringing simple, high-quality ingredients together with a fundamental fueling thought process offers fuel to sustain health and performance, and leaves time to do what makes you feel most like you—run.

The aim of *Finish Line Fueling* is to inspire ditching the pre-packed foods and performance products laced with less ideal ingredients. Emphasis is placed on a simple whole food grocery list packed with essential nutrients every caliber runner requires to thrive. Focusing on whole food, nutrient dense ingredients allows for a healthy, high performance regimen to unfold and open the door to many aspects of a good quality life.

Fundamental Fuel

Are there goals you strive for when you put together a meal or snack? What do you want to achieve from your plate? Some runners reach for favorite and routine comfort foods because it offers a sense of security in weight management and predictability. Other runners yearn to fill a void response to cravings and overwhelming hunger. Sometimes simply working in a quality source protein or having a vegetable land on the plate feels like blue ribbon kind of meal.

Think of fueling the mind, palate, and body in support of health, performance, and overall quality of life. What we feel like consuming can often be driven by factors beyond taste or "good" and "bad" food choices.

Consider a runner who eats very little fat. This naturally creates an urge, and maybe even sense of anxiety, to consume a very fatty meal because the body sends a strong enough message to answer the fat discrepancy. By consuming a small source of fat with meals and snacks as often as possible, the runner will feel more at peace while satisfying the palate and body. The more one can identify with what the body needs, the more one can appropriately respond without going to extremes.

The monitoring of calories-in and calories-out plays a major role in weight management, race weight, and overall health. However, the foundation of a true high quality diet can be lost with calorie-driven fueling; it can also instigate a negative food relationship with thoughts of feeling "good" or "bad" about eating. A shift in focus should be to achieve target ranges of macronutrients—carbohydrates, protein, and fat—in meeting individual nutrition needs. This offers a spirit of "fueling," not just eating.

It's essential for a runner to develop a base understanding of macronutrient needs as they relate to individual weight, training, and overall life goals. This will be a tremendous help to understanding what type of balance your body needs in the day between food groups as well as fueling great training and racing. Knowing the body requires 400 grams of carbohydrates a day, yet realizing an average day holds around 250 grams of carbohydrates offers the opportunity to gradually adjust the diet and better sustain needs.

While it's advantageous to gain understanding in target macronutrient goals, over-calculating food can be overwhelming to many runners. This is especially true when labels are not present or life gets hectic. To limit the number of variables in analyzing what the body needs, support decision making at meals, and find a balance between life and meeting macronutrient goals, I encourage a concept called fundamental fueling. Fundamental fueling is the basic goal a runner should strive for at meals and snacks as often as possible. It supports hitting daily target nutrient needs, and minimizes nutrient deficits and eating extremes, while optimizing health and performance.

There are five key components to focus on as the basis of fundamental fueling. The objective is to be aware of each component and their source at meals and snacks. When a runner focuses on these five components at meals and snacks as often as possible, nutrient goals for the day are much more likely to come together in an ideal fashion. It takes the stress out of hitting a daily grand total number by breaking mealtime into smaller parts. It simplifies performance fueling and a well-balanced diet.

The five key components are to 1) consume a source of quality carbohydrates that contains fiber; 2) eat lean protein; 3) eat healthy fat; 4) enhance meals with colorful anti-oxidant-rich foods such as fruits and vegetables; and 5) be sure to drink enough fluid to maintain hydration.

5 Key Fundamental Fueling Components

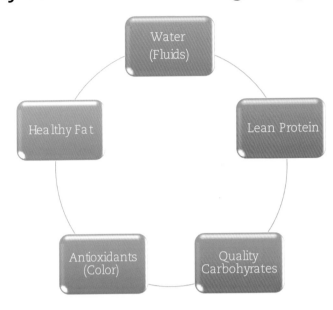

*** Strive to consume a source of each of the five fundamental fueling components at meals and snacks as often as possible. ***

There are a lot of powerful foods to choose from with fundamental fueling, but no single food is "super" enough to single out as the ideal single source of nutrition. It is easy to be coaxed into thinking a single food or ingredient can heal all wounds. As with all forms of life, balance is required. Striving for balance through many different high quality food sources daily is ideal.

The learning curve of putting together a meal that contains a source of quality carbohydrates, lean protein, healthy fat, antioxidants, and water comes with a basic understanding of what the sources of these components are. It is very easy for one or more of the components to slip through the cracks.

Consider a meal of grilled chicken over a bed of green leafy vegetables and topped with low fat salad dressing. Sounds "healthy," but this meal does not offer fundamental fueling balance. As the day continues, discrepancy in fuel sources compound and over time can contribute to nutrient inadequacies and hard to suppress cravings.

The same "healthy" meal becomes more balanced using a fundamental fuel philosophy by eating a bed of green leafy vegetables topped with grilled chicken, avocado, white beans, and fresh fruit. The meal reaches a whole new level in terms of "healthy." Chicken and beans serve as protein sources, avocado supplies healthy fat, and the beans and fruit serve as quality carbohydrate sources. A colorful plate suggests an array of powerful antioxidants. Drinking water, milk, or juice with the meal supports hydration.

Water (Fluids)	• Water, dairy and non-dairy milk, kefir, kombucha, ginger tea, green tea, black tea, and chamomile tea, tart cherry juice, orange juice, grapefruit juice
Lean Protein	• Chicken, salmon, bass, shrimp, scallops, tuna, black cod, rainbow trout, mussels, halibut, lean beef, lean pork, egg, milk, cheese, yogurt, black beans, garbanzo beans, kidney beans, lentils, black-eyed peas, pinto beans, quinoa, hemp seed, tofu, green peas, tempeh, nuts and seeds
Quality Carbohydrates	• Sweet and white potato, rutabaga, turnip, beet, parsnip, quinoa, brown rice, oatmeal, fruit, corn, popcorn, buckwheat, beans, wild rice, brown rice, rice cakes, milk, yogurt, whole grain bread, pasta, and cereal
Antioxidants (Color)	• Blueberry, strawberry, cranberry, raspberry, plum, cherry, orange, mango, peach, apricot, cantaloupe, kiwi, watermelon, pineapple, pear, broccoli, asparagus, avocado, beet, tomato, sweet potato, spinach, kale, carrot, winter squash, bell pepper, squash, beans, nuts and seeds, spices, tea
Healthy Fat	• Fatty fish, flax, hemp, chia, and pumpkin seed, avocado, extra virgin olive oil, high oleic safflower oil, walnut, almond, hazelnut, pistachio, coconut, as well as real butter and ghee in moderation.

Macronutrient is a term to describe carbohydrates, protein, and fat. The three macronutrients serve as fuel for the body in meeting energy needs in the form of calories. A balance between carbohydrates, protein, and fat is essential for health, weight management, and performance. While every athlete should strive for the balance of macronutrients, all too often runners place great emphasis on a single macronutrient for weight management purposes and neglect a healthy balance of macronutrients. While heading down this weight management and isolated macronutrient path, the idea of achieving necessary micronutrients beyond iron and calcium is disregarded.

Micronutrient is the term for the substances and chemicals, such as vitamins and minerals, required in small amounts that allow the body to perform normal processes. I lump micronutrients into the category of antioxidants to simplify the fundamental fueling concept; however, the broad category of micronutrients entails more than just antioxidants. Focusing on antioxidants in terms of color is a great starting place. The more colorful a meal or snack, the more likely one is to achieve a broad range of micronutrients. Examples of micronutrients are iron, calcium, potassium, zinc, vitamin K, and magnesium. Foods that are high in micronutrients are considered good quality and dense in nutrients.

Questions may remain in understanding why we need to eat certain foods, what sources are high quality, when do we eat, and how much is needed to offer the most benefits. The below sections will hopefully help.

Carbohydrates: Why, What, When, and How Much?

WHY Carbohydrates?

Carbohydrate availability plays a major role in a runner's ability to sustain an intense training load and perform well in competition. Carbohydrates are the most efficient way for the body to break down energy in the form of glucose to be used by working muscles and the brain. The body stores carbohydrates in the liver as glycogen. When the blood supply of glucose is depleted, the liver is responsible for converting glycogen to glucose as a fuel source. If there is not enough glycogen stored or if stored glycogen is depleted during a long or intense training session, a source of fast absorbing carbohydrate, such as sports drink or energy gel, is useful in replenishing blood glucose and sustaining performance.

Depletion of carbohydrates is a major cause of fatigue during exercise. Optimizing the carbohydrate status of the body can minimize fatigue. The longer and more intense the exercise, the more important it is to consume adequate carbohydrates in the diet.

WHAT Carbohydrate Sources?

It is important to think of carbohydrates in terms of quality. Reducing, if not eliminating, candy or cookies makes more sense than cutting fresh fruit, brown rice, sweet potato, or whole grain pasta. Runners often justify sweets, but find it no problem to cut quality carbohydrates. The better quality choices consistently made in the diet, the more likely required nutrients to maintain good health and performance can be achieved.

Most often a runner should reach for natural forms of quality carbohydrates that are processed as little as possible. Quality, slow carbohydrates typically contain fiber, are absorbed more slowly, and contain a greater amount of nutrients. Many of these foods can be prepared in bulk and stored in the freezer or refrigerator for use like many of the convenience foods that line the shelf, yet aren't laced undesirable ingredients.

Great carbohydrate sources include: sweet potatoes, brown rice, beans and lentils, fresh and dried fruit, oat and oat bran, quinoa, barley, whole grain wheat germ or bran, spelt, corn, peas, and white potato.

Under certain training and racing circumstances various forms of sugar, or fast carbohydrates, will serve as a rapid fuel source. Fast carbohydrates are necessary because they enter the blood stream quickly and support fueling goal performance. Examples of common fast carbohydrates are sports drinks, dried fruit, sports gels, honey, sport jellybeans, and maple syrup. Figuring out what source of carbohydrate is best tolerated during training sessions will help runners support a solid race day plan.

Outside of training windows and racing, many of the fast sugar sources should be limited. Take for instance an opportunity to eat Greek yogurt with fresh fruit and granola instead of yogurt made with sugar syrup and outdone with food-dye laden candy toppings. Natural forms of sugar such as those present in milk and fruit are beneficial to a healthy diet. Consuming high quantities of sugar in processed foods can contribute to a diet low in nutrients and increase risk of inflammation.

WHEN to Consume Carbohydrates

Daily Needs

The number of carbohydrate grams a runner needs daily varies significantly based on activity level, age, weight, medical history, and more. There is no one-size-fits-all in meeting carbohydrate goals. With that in mind, a carb-free diet is not recommended. There may be stories of the runner who ran endlessly for hours on low or no carbohydrates, but this is not the best strategy for a training runner who desires to maximize their personal performance.

Low or no carbohydrates may work for a short time, but eventually the discrepancy in fuel can compound, as will the stressors on the body. Chronic low carbohydrate dieting for heavily training runners can snowball to ups and downs in body weight, insufficient calories and nutrients, depleted immune function, increased injury risk, and even the potential for overtraining syndrome. Very low volume beginner runners may feel sufficiently fueled with a lower carbohydrate approach, but as training requirements increase, so do carbohydrate requirements.

Slow carbohydrates should make up most of the carbohydrates in the diet, and be part of meals and snacks as often as possible. Consume quality carbohydrates in frequent doses. Including carbohydrates often throughout the day allows a runner greater opportunity to hit target goals by the end of the day instead of cramming as many carbohydrates as possible into a single meal. Spacing carbohydrates throughout the day also offers the body greater ability to manage the carbohydrate load which supports healthy digestion, blood sugar control, and consistent energy levels.

The more often a runner makes an effort to consume high quality carbohydrates at meals and snacks, the less likely they will feel the urge to binge on a sleeve of cookies or fall into the evening bowl of ice cream routine. Craving sweets in general may be the body communicating that a diet is low in sufficient quality carbohydrates. Be sure quality carbohydrates are a priority at meals and snacks.

Training and Competition Needs

When to consume carbohydrates relative to training can become somewhat strategic. To narrow how carbohydrates should be used in training, remember three key windows: 1) carbohydrates should be consumed as part of the pre-run meal, 2) during training and racing sessions lasting greater than 60 to 90 minutes, and 3) within about 30 minutes after long, challenging, or glycogen depleting efforts.

Fast carbohydrates are quick to absorb by the body and a beneficial source of fuel during training and racing sessions lasting greater than 60 to 90 minutes, when glycogen stores can become depleted. Fast carbohydrate sources can be beneficial before or after training or racing sessions if a runner's appetite is low and consumption of adequate carbohydrates to fuel performance or recovery is difficult. A drizzle of honey into a bowl of oats before a race can support a runner who is too nervous to eat their carbohydrate goal with bulky foods. Chocolate milk after a workout is another example of a source of quick carbohydrates that supports refueling the athlete with a poor post-workout appetite for solid foods.

Fast absorbing carbohydrates work well for training purposes before, during, and after exercise. Outside of training, the majority of carbohydrates consumed in the diet should be in the form of slow carbohydrates.

HOW MUCH Carbohydrate?

Carbohydrates should always be an emphasis of meals and snacks. How many grams of carbohydrate a runner consumes in a day largely depends on the level of activity. The more active a runner, the more carbohydrate intake increases. Activity level refers to more than just how many hours a week a runner trains. The runner who sits the majority of the day with a desk job will likely require the lower end of the carbohydrate range based on training compared to the runner who is constantly walking or heavy lifting throughout the day.

Daily Goals:
5 to 6 g/kg for runners training less than an hour several days/week

6 to 7 g/kg for runners training about 1 hour/day

7 to 8 g/kg for runners training just over an hour/day

8 to 9 g/kg for runners training up to 2 hours/day

10 to 12 g/kg for runners training greater than 2 hours/day

Performance Goals

Before exercise, consider a starting point to consume roughly 40 to 60 grams of carbohydrate per hour before a workout or race. This will enforce the idea that the closer you eat to exercise, the less you want to eat. The longer from exercise a meal or snack is consumed, the more eaten. Such a concept allows a runner to feel light, digested, and fast on their feet. The aim is to feel satisfied, but not heavy with food by the time the run starts.

After implementing the early 40 to 60 g/hour concept a runner should train the gut in finding their personal "sweet spot." A highly competitive runner will want to train to gut and pre-run nerves, and eat as much as half of their body weight in grams of carbohydrate per hour that they eat before a race starts.

Consider this application in terms of the late day run. A runner leaving the office after a long workday with early signs of hunger, yet needing to begin a workout in less than an hour can apply this model. A snack of a large piece of fruit and serving of buckwheat oat granola would offer the runner about 240 calories, 4 g of fat, 45 to 55 g of carbs, and 5 to 6 g of protein. A nice combination and enough time to feel light and digested if consumed about 30 to 60 minutes before a run.

During long or hard training sessions, as well as races lasting greater than 60 to 90 minutes, effort should be made to consume fast carbohydrates. A rate of about 30 to as much as 90 grams of carbohydrate broken up over the course of each hour is ideal. A mid-range of 45 to 70 grams of carbohydrate per hour often works well as a starting goal and can be adjusted up or down slightly based on tolerance and preferences. When a runner exceeds about 55 to 60 grams of carbohydrate per hour, it is best if carbohydrates are from a combination of glucose and fructose sources.

Think of fueling during performance as a slow intravenous flow of steady nutrition that will support maximum performance. Develop a routine to consume fuel at regular intervals throughout the run. Explore more specifics on race strategy in Section 4.

The more mileage and demanding training a runner puts in, the more recovery nutrition needs to be a priority. A runner who takes a day off between each run likely has enough time to restock glycogen stores. The runner with two or more workouts a day will benefit from refueling within 30 minutes of each effort. Refueling with about half of body weight in grams of carbohydrates, paired with 10 to 30 grams of protein, would be ideal. Follow this post-run snack with a meal within 1 to 2 hours.

Protein: Why, What, When, and How Much?

WHY Eat Protein?

Protein is made up of important building blocks called amino acids that are required for tissue repair, growth, essential hormones, digestive enzymes, neurotransmitters, antibodies to fight infection, and more. This vital source of energy provides the necessary building blocks required to manage the constant breakdown and synthesis of protein. The body can produce some amino acids, while others must be consumed through diet.

All amino acids play important roles in the body. For instance, glutamine is an abundant amino acid in the body. When glutamine status is compromised runners are more susceptible to reduced immune function, slow recovery, poor performance, and increased gut permeability. While glutamine is essential for a training runner, a balance of all amino acids is required for optimal performance and health.

A deficiency of protein puts a runner at risk for muscle and general weakness, frequent illnesses, anemia, and increase risk of overtraining syndrome. While carbohydrates are essential to support blood glucose and glycogen stores, carbohydrates paired with protein is most effective at aiding a solid training regimen.

WHAT Sources of Protein?

Healthy whole foods sources of protein should be the emphasis of every athlete. Foods rich in protein include: turkey, chicken, beef, pork, eggs, seafood, beans and lentils, dairy, quinoa, amaranth, teff, peas, soy (such as tofu and tempeh), shelled pumpkin seeds, hemp seeds, and nuts. Rotate protein sources often, aiming for a variety of power-supporting nutrition.

If a specialized diet requires limiting a large group of protein dense foods, it is very important to make a list and develop a plan to replace the undesirable protein with sources that fit into the runner's diet. A vegan runner who excludes all forms of animal protein will want to ensure the diet is rich with a variety of non-animal protein sources as well as ingredients that support sufficient B12 intake.

Protein supplements can be used to occasionally fill macronutrient gaps, but should not to replace whole food meals. Protein supplements should complement great fueling, not replace quality whole food meals.

WHEN to Consume Protein

A great rule of thumb is to make an effort to consume protein with meals and snacks as often as possible. Incorporating protein in small frequent doses spread throughout the day is most effective compared to eating one large dose at a single meal. Eating a moderate amount of protein divided among all meals and snacks supports protein synthesis and the likelihood of consuming sufficient protein in the day. Make sure protein is a part of pre-run and recovery fueling.

A very small amount of protein may support performance during exercise, but including protein during exercise is often poorly tolerated. A runner participating in very long event, such as an ultra-running event, will want to test the amount and source of lean protein that is well-tolerated while running. Even during a long event, protein consumption should be small and steady. Sufficient carbohydrates should be the primary focus throughout the event to support gastric emptying.

HOW MUCH Protein?

If the aim to eat protein at meals and snacks is applied, there is less concern over the grand total of protein at the end of the day. Consuming two to three meals a day with close to 30 grams of protein and two to three snacks with 10 to 20 grams of protein would successfully meet the needs of many runners. The meal or snack before and after training should contain roughly 10 to 30 grams of a protein.

Protein needs should be heightened for about the first two weeks of a new training regimen or for the first two weeks of any increase in training load. This can be as simple as increasing the serving size just slightly at meals, snacks, and after training sessions. Weight-loss seeking runners training with a reduced energy intake will want to consume as much as 2 grams of protein per kilogram to prevent muscle loss.

Protein Goals:

Daily

Most runners should consume 1.2 to 2.0 grams of protein per kilogram of body weight. If calculating kilograms gets tricky, multiply your weight by 0.6 to 0.9 to offer a protein target range. The heavier training runner would require the upper end of the target range, while a lower mileage runner will require the low end.

Before, During, and After Exercise

Aim for about 10 to 30 grams of protein before and after exercise. Most often during exercise very little or no protein is required. A small, steady protein intake during a long event such as ultra-races is beneficial.

The more demanding the training regimen, the greater the protein needs.

Fat: Why, What, When, and How Much?

WHY Eat Fat

Fat is an extremely important part of a healthy diet. Fat is needed for growth and development, to transport fat-soluble vitamins, has hormone-like components, cushions organs, and can protect against disease. There are health supporting forms of fat and health limiting forms of fat. Consumption of healthy forms of fat will support overall health and reduce inflammation.

WHAT Sources of Fat?

Unsaturated fats in the form of monounsaturated or polyunsaturated are a healthy form of fat to include in the diet. They are primarily found in vegetable products like olive oil, high oleic safflower oil, walnuts, olives, wheat germ, and avocados. A balance of omega-3 and omega-6 essential fatty acids is also very important in the diet. Essential fatty acids are influential in times of inflammation. Sources of essential fatty acids are fish, pumpkin seeds, walnuts, flaxseed, chia seeds, hemp seeds, egg yolk, and green leafy vegetables.

Saturated and trans fats are to be limited or avoided altogether in the diet. A diet with about 10 percent or less of total fat from saturated fat is considered healthy. There is no safe level of trans fat. A runner's diet should consist of 20 to 30 percent of total calories from fat as part of a healthy diet. Compare food labels or research ingredients for fat sources to allow for healthier food choices and greater consumption of the "good" fats.

WHEN to Consume Fat

There are some key thoughts to consider when it comes to the timing and amount of fat consumed. To keep in line with the fundamental fueling thought process, a small to moderate amount of fat with each meal will promote a sense of satisfaction with meals and spread the fat load evenly throughout the day.

There's no question a runner requires fat, but fat can interfere with the ability to consume enough carbohydrates and protein. Since carbohydrates are a major fuel source for runners, the amount and timing of fat should be considered. When fat dominates a meal, "room" for carbohydrates can diminish. The aim is to find a balance between consuming enough healthy fat to meet daily requirements and taste preferences, yet leave room for optimizing carbohydrate and protein needs.

A pre-run or pre-race meal should be low in fat with emphasis on carbohydrates as well as a source of protein. Fat is slow to digest. If too much fat is consumed with this meal there is an increase in potential to suffer from gastrointestinal distress on the run. Nut butters, avocado, and touch of healthy oils can still work into a pre-race meal, but used as a thin spread or light topping.

The day or two before a long event such as a marathon or ultra-race consider low-fat thinking the entire day. This allows for any fat calories to be replaced by glycogen-stocking carbohydrate calories. For example, a turkey sandwich normally topped with fat sources such as mayonnaise, cheese, and avocado would shift to a turkey sandwich topped with fresh tomato, lettuce, and mustard. The fat calories from the mayo, cheese, and avocado toppings would transfer to an extra serving of fruit, low fat crackers, or baked potato. Once the race is complete, the runner can go back to regularly spacing normal fat intake throughout the day.

HOW MUCH Fat to Consume?

Generally a runner would first meet protein and carbohydrate needs. Remaining calories would be in the form of fat to meet total energy needs. Another guide is to shoot for just under half of body weight in grams of fat per day. This can adjust slightly up or down based on training demands and calorie needs. A very high mileage runner may need to consume their full body weight in grams of fat daily to maintain weight.

Daily Fat Goal

Just under half of body weight in grams of fat daily, adjusting up or down based on training demands and calorie needs.

Fat is not required during competition, unless in very small amounts for satiety reasons during a very long event such as an ultra-race.

While focusing on the key concepts of fundamental fueling, I encourage you to listen to your body and respond accordingly. This is where things can get tricky. As runners we are often suppressing physical cues, such as fatigue and discomfort. The exact opposite is true with fueling. The body is often trying to communicate need. For example, a constant craving for sweets may suggest the body is really asking for more quality carbohydrates from the diet. Desire for salty chips or pretzels may suggest a need for electrolytes and fluids.

Applying the concept of fundamental fueling combined with staying in tune to what the body communicates will energize performance and quality of life.

Light Snack—30–60 Minutes Before Run

- Piece of Fruit and Cheese Stick
- 1 c. Whole Grain Dry Cereal
- ½ c. Oatmeal
- Tortilla with ½–1 tbsp. Peanut Butter
- 1 Small Sweet Potato, 1 tbsp. Almond Butter
- Slice of Whole Grain Toast with Sliced Fruit and 2 tbsp. Yogurt
- ½ c. Yogurt with ½ c. Granola
- ¾ c. Brown Rice and 1 oz. grilled chicken
- 1 Slice Whole Grain Bread, 1–2 oz. Lean Deli Turkey, Mustard

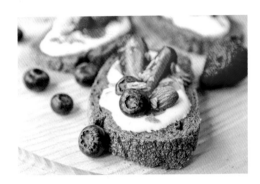

Heavy Snack—60–90 Minutes Before Run

- Cup of Fruit, Cheese Stick, Granola Bar
- 1½ c. Whole Grain dry cereal, 2 tbsp. Nuts, ¼ c. Dried Fruit
- ½ Oatmeal, ½ c Yogurt, ½ c. Fresh Fruit
- Medium Tortilla, 1 tbsp. Peanut Butter, Banana
- 2 oz. Tuna, 20–30 Whole Grain Crackers, Piece of Fruit
- Peanut Butter and Jelly Sandwich, Yogurt
- Medium Sweet Potato, ¼ c. Yogurt, ¼ c. Granola
- 1 c. Brown Rice, 2 oz. grilled chicken, piece of fruit
- 2 Slices Whole Grain Bread, 2 oz. Lean Deli Turkey, Tomato, Mustard

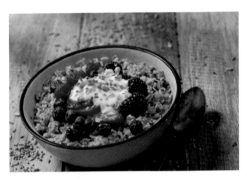

Light Meal—90–120 Minutes Before Run

- Piece of Fruit, Whole Grain Bagel, Slice of Cheese, Granola Bar
- 2 c. Whole Grain Cereal, 1 c. Milk, Banana
- ¾ c. Oatmeal, ½ c. Yogurt, 1–2 tbsp. Raisins, Cup of Fruit
- 1 Large Tortilla, 1–2 tbsp. Peanut Butter, 1 Banana, 1 tbsp. Honey
- Peanut Butter and Jelly Sandwich, Piece of Fruit, Cup of Milk
- 2 oz. Chicken, Large Baked Sweet Potato, Piece of Fruit, ¼ c. Yogurt
- 1¼ c. Brown Rice, ½ c. peas, 2 oz. Grilled Chicken, Piece of Fruit
- 2 oz. Tuna, Cup of Noodles, Cup of Fruit, Granola Bar
- 2 Slices Whole Grain Bread, 2 oz. Lean Deli Turkey, Tomato, Mustard, Piece of Fruit, Granola Bar

—Find Your Fit—

Test the food sources and volume you tolerate best with basic *starting* guidelines:

Before Exercise: Begin with 40–60 grams of carbohydrate with a source of protein per hour before exercise.

Example: Test 50–90 grams carbohydrate and 10–20 grams protein for a meal 90 minutes before exercise.

Fluids—Drink in effort to achieve light-colored urine prior to exercise start.

Avoid Monotony

In many ways, it makes sense to eat what makes you feel good, supports maintenance of a healthy weight, and promotes consistency in terms of what to expect during a workout. On the other hand, food monotony may not offer sufficient nutrient diversity and can lead to insufficiencies that interfere with health and performance. This is particularly the case if one eats the exact same, low nutrient or calorie restrictive foods daily.

Although a runner who eats the same thing every day may make "healthy" choices, the runner's choices may consistently lack a nutrient such as zinc. Over time a chronic low zinc intake interferes with tissue repair and frequent injuries. Insufficient zinc can also impair immune function leading to frequent battles with colds and sicknesses. Gut permeability and related food sensitivities can be associated with a low zinc status. Diet diversity offers the body greater opportunity to achieve all of the nutrients needed to support health and performance.

The recipes available in *Finish Line Fueling* primarily stem from one main grocery list. A nice diversity in foods and broad range of nutrients can be accomplished within the one grocery list. This maintains a sense of comfort in eating within a similar spectrum of foods, yet offers nutrient quality a runner needs to thrive.

To deter from a very specific, mundane food routine, consider implementing a minimum three-day rotation of meals with the goal to vary food sources. The rotation can still be somewhat regimented within the three to five day timeframe, if desired, but maintain diversity within the three to five day span. An easy way to make this happen is to generate a list of your three favorite breakfasts, three favorite post-workout snacks or meals, three favorite lunches, and three favorite dinners.

A fantastic starting point in gaining a better understanding of your general micronutrient intake is to log a few days at a time in the smartphone app or web-based program called Cronometer. Knowing how many calories are consumed versus burned may come in handy at times, but Cronometer is a tool to focus on how to maximize micronutrients within overall macronutrient goals. When athletes focus on macronutrients and micronutrients performance goals are optimized and consistent.

Breakfast rotation ideas:
1. Quinoa power bowl and fresh fruit.
2. Almond granola sweet potato and cup of juice.
3. Savory maca oats, fresh fruit, cup of kefir.

Lunch rotation ideas:
1. Turkey Reuben with low fat milk, kale chips, and fresh fruit.
2. Southwest sweet potato salad, cup of milk, and stuffed dates.
3. Chicken and white bean salad with spelt pita bread and fresh fruit.

Dinner rotation ideas:

1. Pumpkin chili over noodles and fresh fruit.
2. All-in-one meatloaf muffins, mashed potatoes, side salad, fresh fruit.
3. Baked salmon steak with spinach and mushrooms, brown rice, and fresh fruit.

Snack rotation ideas for each day:

1. Fruit on the bottom yogurt and granola, energy bar and fresh fruit, oat-mega cookies and milk.
2. Toasted grain bread with hummus, tomato, and nutritional yeast, chocolate pudding topped with fresh banana.
3. Bran flakes cereal with milk and fresh fruit, cherry banana cooler, and a granola bar.

Cronometer is one of a few food tracking applications that offers a guide in tracking micronutrients. If a trend of low zinc intake is observed after tracking for a week in Cronometer, greater effort should be made in increasing daily food sources of zinc. Cronometer is a great tool for runners to appreciate the nutrient density of a diet they are consuming.

The goal is always to maximize nutrients through a whole food diet as often as possible. Supplements may be required to address insufficiencies; however, a whole food, nutrient-rich diet should be the main priority.

Daily Fluids and Electrolytes

Health and hydration go hand-in-hand. Proper hydration is essential for the body to function normally, let alone handle a high level training. Fluid goals in terms of performance can be found in the Race Strategy section, beginning on page 45. Generally the guideline for daily hydration assessment is to achieve and maintain light-colored urine throughout the day. However, consider evaluating daily hydration beyond urine color.

Morning Weight

Measuring your morning weight can be a great way to assess daily fluid balance. This is your weight first thing in the morning after using the restroom, but before eating or drinking, and always dressed in same amount of clothing.

A runner may not have rehydrated well from the previous day's workout if there is a significant drop in weight one from one day to the next. Compare any morning weight changes with urine color. If weight dropped and urine color is dark, increased effort with hydration should be implemented. This can guide the 5 a.m.

run. Going into a workout with a drop in weight and dark urine may not make for the best workout. It may be worth running later in the day or running a route with access to fluids during the run.

Fluid Choices

Water is the primary fluid source that should be consumed most often throughout the day. If the diet trends more toward coffee and soda than water, the diet needs revamping. Most often I recommend a sixteen to twenty-swallow guideline versus a specific number of ounces to drink in a day. The swallow guideline allows room for the body to regulate fluid needs. Filling the mouth with twenty gulps of water, such as after a dehydrating run, will offer about 20 ounces. Sipping sixteen swallows of water offers roughly 8 ounces of fluid.

The swallow guideline is to drink sixteen to twenty swallows of water upon waking in the morning, and each time there is a drive to eat or drink. If after sixteen to twenty swallows of water a runner is inclined to still drink more water, coffee, or reach for salty crackers, then he or she will be able to better determine why they are reaching for the food or drink. Often runners reach for salty foods and less than ideal beverages because a true thirst is not addressed. This guideline supports healthy hydration, while still allowing the body to decipher fluid needs.

Salt

I often add salt in my cooking without reservation. A diet low in processed foods and rich in whole food will naturally be low sodium. An athlete who follows a primarily whole food diet will require adding salt in order to meet electrolyte needs. A high sweat loss runner with a heavy training load will require more sodium than a low mileage, low sweat loss runner. Add or reduce salt to taste in the recipes here based on your drive to consume sodium and training regimen.

A runner who is making the transition to whole foods, yet still consumes a significant amount of convenient foods, dines out frequently, or has been diagnosed with a medical condition that requires a low sodium diet may need to be more cautious with their sodium intake.

Consider choosing salt that contains trace minerals such as magnesium, copper, zinc, and iodine. Real, Himalayan, or Celtic sea salts are a few examples.

Quick Tips:

- Aim for a balance of quality carbohydrates with fiber paired with a source of lean protein, a small source of healthy fat, and colorful ingredients at meals and snacks as often as possible.

- Focus on macronutrients—carbohydrates, protein, and fat—instead of counting calories.

- Create a rotation of quality food sources versus eating the exact same foods each day.

- Drink sixteen to twenty swallows of water before meals, snacks, and each urge to drink a beverage other than water.

- Add quality salt to foods often if the diet is minimally processed.

- Use a food tracking system that tracks micronutrients, such as Cronometer, for about three to seven days to gain a better understanding of average micronutrient intake trends.

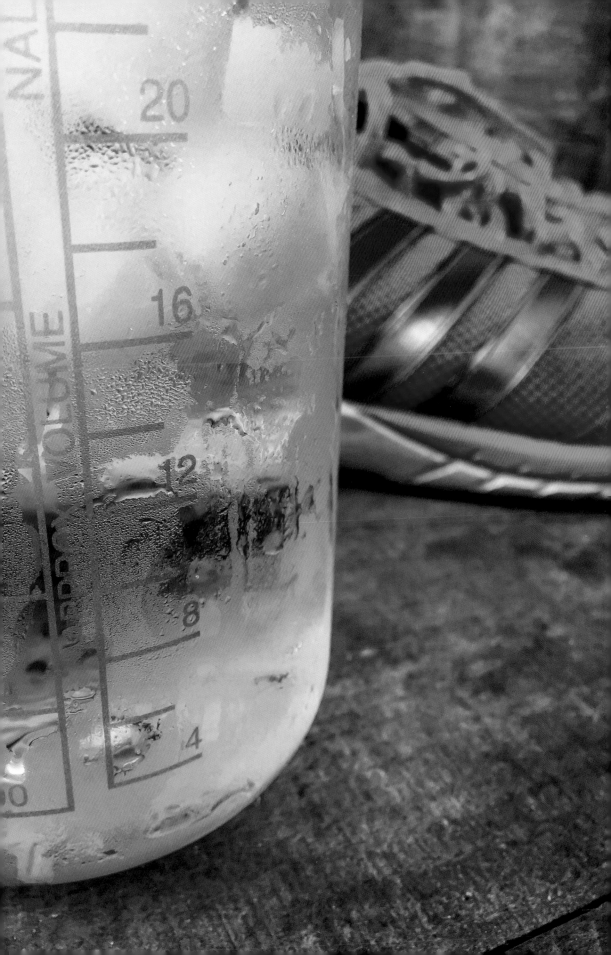

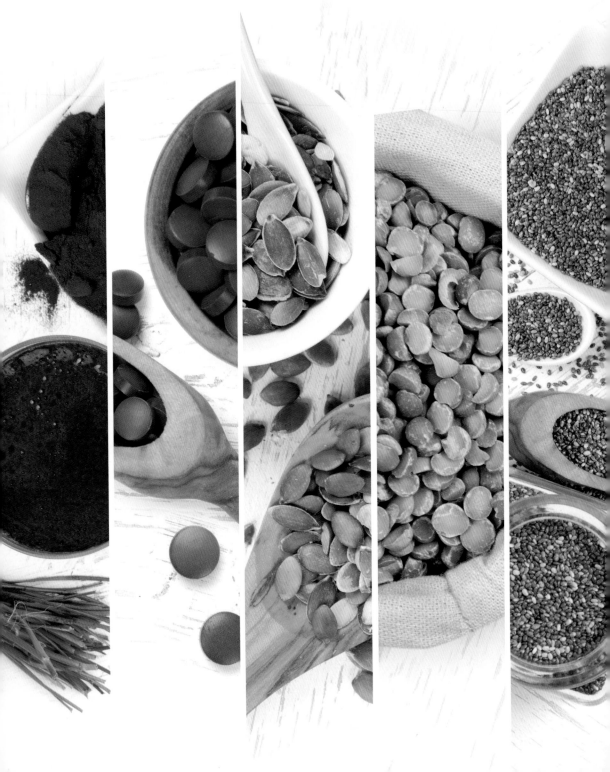

FEED THE IMMUNE SYSTEM

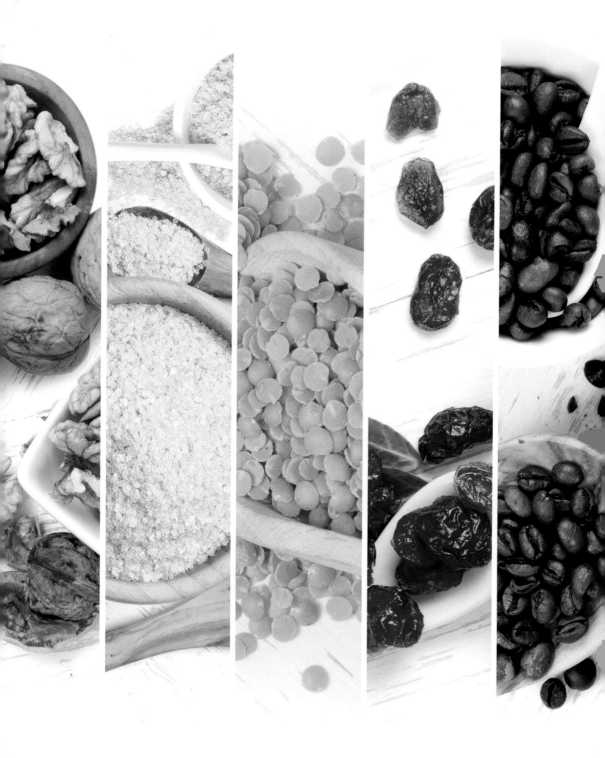

The number of hours of sleep per day, work stress load, training load, body weight, and nutritional balance can all affect how well the body functions. If one or more of these variables is out of balance, a snowball effect can induce depletion, poor training and performance, a decline in overall health, and even contribute to chronic disease. Nutrition is one way to combat stress and depletion. By optimizing food choices and nutrients consumed, the body can better respond stress and support a healthy immune system while maintaining a tough training load.

The most common cause of an upper respiratory tract infection in athletes is a depleted immune system. After working with many athletes, I have gained a much deeper appreciation for various symptoms endurance athletes may experience related to stress load and how the immune system responds. As these symptoms compound, the more an athlete is likely to feel performance limitations, and even a decline in quality of life. Symptoms include:

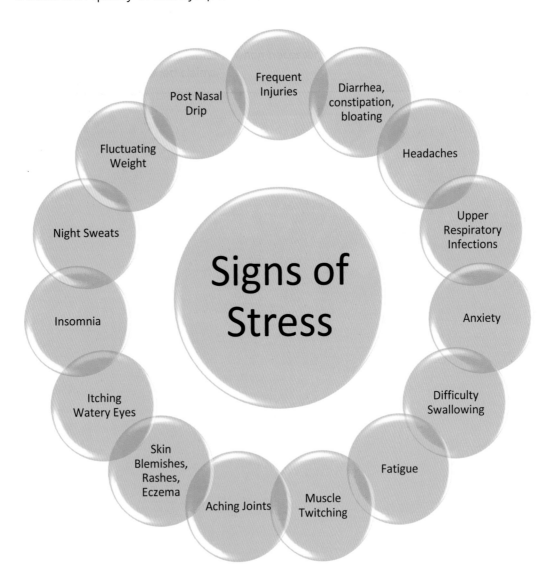

Finish Line Fueling

Overcoming Stress and Depletion

Many athletes are familiar with general guidelines to support minimizing symptoms of an overactive immune system. Common recommendations include avoiding over training, consuming sufficient calories, monitoring morning heart rate trends, and striving for sufficient sleep. Such strategy is applied in an effort to minimize inflammation and the risk of a seasonal cold setback. A runner's nutrition strategy can also take a broader approach to overcoming stress and depletions. Integrating probiotics, choosing food with low inflammatory ingredients, and eating an overall high quality diet can support calming the immune system while optimizing recovery and performance.

There is a common misconception that running as many miles as possible at the lowest body weight possible is the key to success. A decline in both health and performance can occur as a result of an inadequate diet at a time when the body is stressed from training and demands calories and nutrients. Proper nutrition is critical to health and performance, yet brushed to the side in favor of calorie control.

Meeting mileage goals and a lean physique will support performance; however, being thin and fast does not mean healthy. There are many facets to good health. Chronically performing while under-fueled can be detrimental to long-term health. An under-fueled body will eventually surrender and cripple in distress. Consuming sufficient calories is one of the first lines of defense for a healthy immune system.

Carbohydrates

Carbohydrates are essential for an athlete with a suppressed immune system. A diet lacking sufficient carbohydrates can cause the body to respond to stress with a release of cortisol. A diet continually low in carbohydrates can lead to muscle breakdown, a decrease in the ability for the muscle to accept glucose, and chronic inflammation. Feed the immune system with plenty of quality sources of carbohydrates.

Probiotics

Probiotics are healthy bacteria that occur naturally in foods such as sauerkraut, kimchi, yogurt, kefir, kombucha, buttermilk, unpasteurized cheese, tempeh, and miso. We are constantly learning about the amazing role probiotics play in support of a healthy gut and immune system, and even more so as they pertain to athletes. What we do know is that probiotics support a healthy gut microbiota. A healthy gut plays a role in stress and inflammatory response, nutrient absorption, mental health, and more.

Signs a runner may benefit from an increase in probiotics include antibiotic use, low vitamin K levels, difficulty achieving a normal B vitamin status, frequent upper respiratory tract infections, gastrointestinal disturbances, frequent cavities, and skin conditions.

Making an effort to expand the palate and working in different probiotic strains through a variety of food sources can help to support healthy gut function and the immune system. Fermented vegetables, including various forms of sauerkraut, come in many great flavors. I love snacking on a salty horseradish or dill pickle flavored kraut as a post-run salty, electrolyte replacing side. A heap of flavored kraut or kimchi makes a delicious salad dressing substitute or sandwich topping. Be creative.

Individual strains aid specific symptoms. Evidence supports that lactobacillus and Bifidobacterium strains are the most effective. Working with a health-care provider to optimize the best strains based on individual symptoms is ideal if one chooses to supplement. For example, specific probiotic strains are beneficial in alleviating diarrhea, while others support reducing the risk of upper respiratory infections. A runner with a specific gastrointestinal complaint would be best served by consuming the probiotic strain specific to the symptoms experienced.

It is possible to experience an increase in symptoms as one increases the intake of probiotics. If this is the case, work probiotics in at a slower rate, increasing your intake as tolerated. These symptoms may be a result of the beneficial changes that occur with shifting from bad bacteria to good bacteria in the gut.

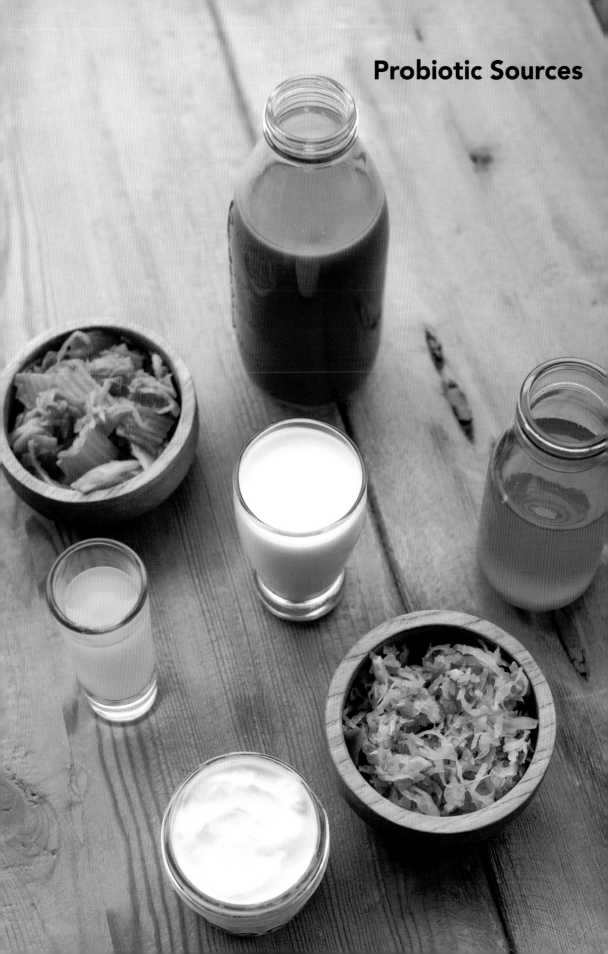

Mindful Ingredients

Could the Food you Eat be a Trigger?

There is no one-size-fits-all when it comes to how the body responds to stress and the immune system. While one runner may find eating an otherwise healthy ingredient such as cinnamon enjoyable, another may experience a runny nose. Runners and other high endurance athletes especially may experience an increase in adverse reactions to the foods they consume; this is directly related to a stressed immune system. Assessing and fueling the body according the how the immune system responds to different foods can be another method to support recovery, performance, and overall health.

It's important that every runner make an effort to gain awareness if the foods consumed induce uncomfortable symptoms. Consider limiting problematic foods from the diet for a few months in an effort to support calming the immune system. As the immune system calms, the more likely inflammatory ingredients can be added back in the future with little to no distress.

The more active the immune system is in regards to symptoms, the more likely there are imbalances in diet, training, and life that need to be addressed. Imbalances can take shape in the form of overtraining, stress load, inadequate calorie intake, sleep, and specific micronutrient insufficiencies. Consider nutrient deficiencies such as B12, zinc, vitamin D, and iron another path of stress the body has to manage. Preventing deficiency lessens the stress load.

The best way to restore and prevent an overactive immune system is to strive for simple, high quality, whole food ingredients. Choosing poor quality foods, such as excess sugar and over processed, chemical laden food, limits nutrient intake and can deplete the body of essential nutrients required for daily functioning let alone demanding training. Making an effort to consume a great whole food diet and correcting any nutrient deficiencies will reduce stress and support calming.

As a general starting point make an effort to incorporate foods rich in immune supporting and anti-inflammatory properties:

- Omega-3 and Oleic Fatty Acids
- Vitamin C
- Zinc
- Vitamin D
- Glutamine

If an immune system is under significant stress, a runner may want to research and discuss other stress reducing options with a health-care professional. Such options include rhodiola, maca root, cordyceps, ginseng, spirulina, and pycnogenol.

Quality over Quantity: Maximize Micronutrients

For runners, numbers are a huge motivation. Weekly mileage goals, splits, personal records, mileage on a pair of shoes, longest run—there are so many ways numbers help drive performance. Attaching numbers to performance as it relates to nutrition can support training, racing, recovery, and overall health.

First, ditch the food tracking systems that focus only on tracking points, calories, and exercise. It is time to take a deeper look at what you are putting into your body. Again, consider Cronometer; among other things, it supports tracking beyond calories and exercise with the capability to track micronutrient trends. While Cronometer may not measure every last milligram of potassium, it is an extremely affordable method for a runner to easily observe and assess general micronutrient trends.

There are two main reasons I recommend this app. First, it drives the desire to choose more nutrient dense food choices. Focusing only on calories may justify reaching for a few pieces of candy if there are calories left at the end of day. However, recognizing a trend of low omega-3 fatty acids may drive a snack of walnuts versus the calorie-driven candy. Cronometer essentially offers a completely different mindset to food choices, unlike the typical calories-in and calories-out recommendations.

Further, Cronometer offers the potential to populate micronutrient trends over a specific timeframe. This offers the potential to be far more proactive with nutrient gaps. A diet chronically low in zinc for a runner can be detrimental in terms of recovery, injury healing and prevention, and gut permeability. If a trend of low zinc is observed, then greater effort should be made in the diet to eat high zinc food sources and to possibly supplement. Once a regimen of maximizing sufficient micronutrients is achieved, tracking can be reduced to periodic reassessment or even eliminated completely.

Taking the concept of micronutrient evaluation a step further, consider testing micronutrients such as zinc, vitamin D, B12, iron, and magnesium as an effective way to support performance and health as well. The Spectracell Micronutrient Test (available with a physician's referral) is a very comprehensive test that supports evaluating vitamins, minerals, amino acids, fatty acids, glucose-insulin interaction, and overall immune system health. Another method of tracking blood analysis is Insider Tracker. It is a resource to assess iron, cortisol, and other inflammatory markers. For a runner, periodically performing such testing could be invaluable tools for performance longevity and overall health. Be sure to discuss any results with your health-care professional to determine the best plan for optimal health.

Eat to Run, Not Run to Eat

Runners are often associated with having a metabolic engine that will burn off any form of fuel as energy supply. When it comes to the immune system, I disagree.

This strategy may be fine as a temporarily means to supply energy, but in the long term, it will not support the health and performance of an athlete who challenges his or her body daily. The idea of metabolic engine may carry some truth if a runner chooses quality fuel, but a runner who frequently dines on lower nutrient foods and a high sugar diet will not have the longevity in sport as would a runner who fuels on quality food choices.

Take for instance a runner who eats a very high carbohydrate diet that is also high in sugar. This is also a runner who dislikes most fruits and vegetables and often struggles to work in protein and fat sources. A high carbohydrate and refined sugar diet contributes to an increase in urinary chromium excretion. This is compounded with any chromium lost through high sweat loss.

Over time, this runner is more likely to experience low chromium due to the combination of chromium lacking in the diet and high chromium loss through secretion. This can be extremely harmful since chromium supports insulin sensitivity and the transport of glucose into cells. This cycle of low chromium intake combined with loss continues and can eventually contribute to poor glucose-insulin interaction, inflammation, slow to heal injuries, and possibly even a diabetic future. Eating well means much more than putting enough calories in the engine.

Quick Tips:
Calm the immune system through simple, whole food ingredients.

- Limit foods that induce uncomfortable symptoms for 3 to 6 months and reintroduce them slowly.
- Assess your micronutrient intake and status through a tracking program such as Cronometer, or via laboratory testing.
- Maximize micronutrients through high quality whole foods and avoid excess empty foods such as processed foods and sugar.
- Reduce stress load with sufficient sleep and appropriate rest in training cycles.
- Consider assessing and increasing whole food intake of zinc, vitamin D, vitamin C, omega-3 fatty acids, glutamine, and probiotics if the immune system is stressed.

Maximize Micronutrient Needs

Calcium

Milk
Yogurt and Kefir
Kale
Broccoli
Cheese
Almonds
Collard Greens
Edamame
Bok Choy
Fortified Orange Juice
Sardines

Zinc

Beef
Mussels, Oysters & Clams
Lamb
Pumpkin Seeds
Sesame Seeds
Lentils
Cashew
Garbanzo Beans
Kefir/Yogurt

Vitamin B12

Beef
Mussels, Oysters & Clams
Salmon
Tuna
Grass-fed Yogurt
Milk
Cheese
Eggs
Nutritional Yeast

Vitamin C

Bell Peppers
Broccoli
Strawberries
Pineapple
Oranges
Kiwi
Cantaloupe
Cauliflower
Spinach
Brussels sprouts

Iron

Grass-fed Beef
Turkey Leg
Lentils
Spinach
Oysters & Clams
Raisins
Blackstrap Molasses
Fortified Cereals
Kidney, Lima, & Navy Beans

Chromium

Broccoli
Barley
Oats
Grape Juice
Orange Juice
Red Wine
Beer
Sweet Potato
Apple
Egg

Magnesium

Pumpkin Seeds
Almonds
Yogurt and Kefir
Avocado
Banana
Spinach
Quinoa
Black and Navy Beans
Cashew

Glutamine

Grass-fed Beef
Bison
Chicken
Eggs
Red Cabbage
Raw Dairy
Spirulina
Cottage Cheese
Wild Caught Fish
Asparagus

Probiotics

Kefir
Yogurt
Cultured Vegetables (Sauerkraut and Kimchi)
Kombucha
Coconut Kefir
Raw cheese
Miso
Sourdough Bread

Sodium

Beets
Celery
Egg
Milk
Cottage Cheese
Yogurt and Kefir
Seaweed
Salmon
Mussels, Oysters, Crab & Lobster

Iodine

Kefir/Yogurt
Cod Fish
Navy Beans
Turkey Breast
Tuna
Eggs
Dried Seaweed
Scallops
Cow's Milk
Salmon

Selenium

Tuna
Halibut, Salmon, Cod
Grass-fed beef
Turkey
Chicken
Egg
Asparagus
Shrimp
Mushroom, Crimini
Brazil Nuts

Vitamin D

Cod Liver Oil
Egg
Fortified Cereal
Fortified Milk
Fortified Orange Juice
Fortified Yogurt
Mackerel
Swiss Cheese
Tuna

Oleic Acid

Avocado
High Oleic Safflower Oil
Olive Oil

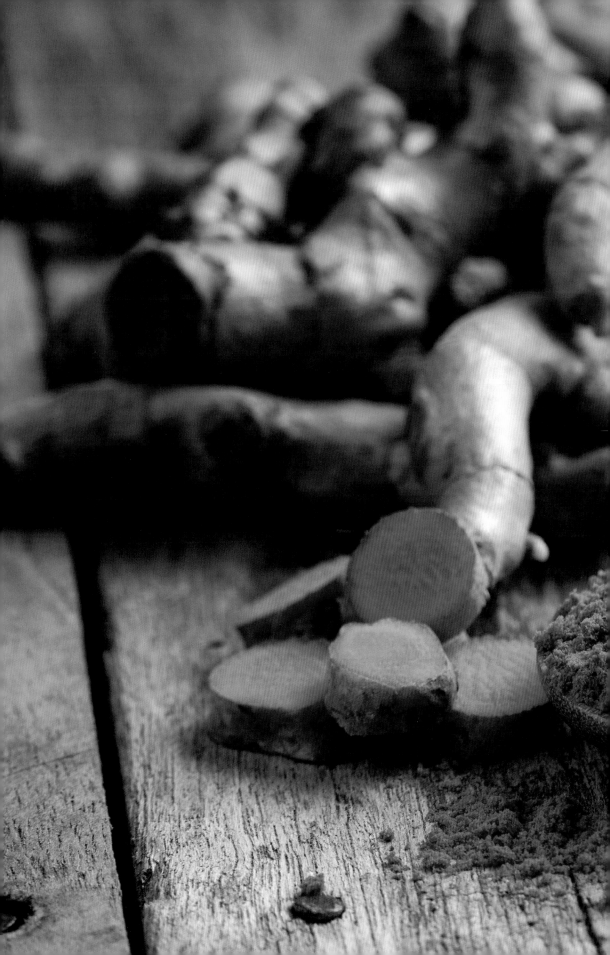

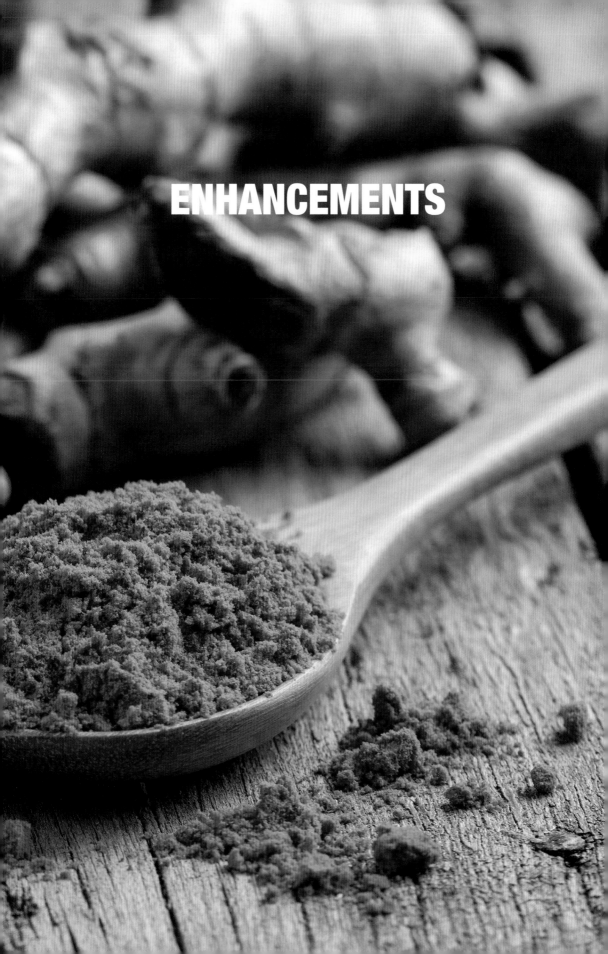

ENHANCEMENTS

Caffeine: When to Use It and When to Lose It

Powering through the final seconds, minutes, and miles of race can be a monumental task. It's usually arduous for the brain to command the legs to maintain speed and postpone exhaustion. Runners who feel they have a positive response to caffeine can take advantage of its ergogenic potential in increasing alertness and decreased perceived level of exertion when running.

The benefit of caffeine in racing shorter distances is less significant than in endurance events, but caffeine can have even mild ergogenic potential for events lasting more than one minute. Because caffeine can enhance alertness, runners who participate in shorter events may find the improved concentration useful in responding to the gun or getting out of start blocks. Contrarily, a nervous response could contribute to a false start.

Application:

Consider limiting daily caffeine use to take advantage of a heightened caffeine response on race day. The less caffeine consumed on a regular basis, the smaller the performance-supporting caffeine dose required on race day. Switch to caffeine-free and decaffeinated beverages during the regular day-to-day. Caffeine can be utilized for specific training circumstances as well as any testing in training to confirm an individual runner's tolerance, sources, and dosing.

Consuming a small dose of caffeine pre-run, yet limiting overall general use of caffeine, may be beneficial in stimulating the bowels and aid a pre-run bowel movement when necessary. This supports performance in minimizing the risk of gastrointestinal upset and a pit stop during the run. Sip just enough caffeinated coffee or tea to stimulate the bowel and then switch to decaffeinated coffee or tea to accomplish limited general caffeine use.

Caffeine takes about an hour to reach a peak, with an effect that can last several hours. Ideally, caffeine would be timed such that performance falls appropriately in this window. An ultra-runner is more likely to benefit from caffeine several hours into a race as compared to a 5K runner who consumes caffeine about an hour before race start.

Caffeine sources can be added to carbohydrate sources throughout a race to support performance for longer distances. The dose necessary to feel the effect depends largely upon general caffeine use and body size. The ideal dose would feel alert and responsive without feeling over stimulated and nervous.

Caffeine also has potential as part of post-workout refueling. When combined with carbohydrates soon after a workout, caffeine supports recovery by replenishing glycogen levels more rapidly. This strategy can be utilized with two-a-day workouts and workouts on consecutive days.

The key with caffeine is to test the best regimen for use based on individual dosing through experimentation in training as well as recovery. If a negative response is experienced, caffeine may not serve an ergogenic role for you. It is important to note that high doses of caffeine are classified as a banned substance by the NCAA. A high dose would be comparable to about 6 to 8 cups of coffee within 2 to 3 hours of competition. This can easily be avoided with the less is more approach described above.

Beets

Yes–beets. While I know many runners would rather eat dirt than acquire a taste for beets, it may just be worth adapting the palate. Beets are a natural source of inorganic nitrate that is converted to nitric oxide. Nitric oxide is a vasodilator that reduces oxygen cost during exercise. This translates to an endurance boosting benefit easily gained by consuming a natural root vegetable.

Application:

The effect of beet juice takes about 2 to 3 hours to peak, which could be well timed with a pre-race breakfast. Research suggests it offers the greatest performance benefit for exercise lasting anywhere from 5 to 30 minutes, but runners of all distances have been known to test the potential endurance boosting benefit of beet juice.

The best way to determine dosing of beet juice is to test it during race-like training conditions. Note that beet juice is likely to briefly change urine color and possibly stool to a pink or red tone. In addition, high doses of beets may induce a gastrointestinal response and urge to use the restroom in some runners. Consider testing the best dose to support performance and limit any potential gastrointestinal setbacks.

Concentrated forms of beet juice are available in shots via the Internet and at local health food stores. A concentrated beet juice shot is often easier for a runner to consume versus drinking 16 ounces of pre-race beet juice. Consider purchasing beet juice shots from organic sources.

Tart Cherry Juice

Tart cherry juice can reduce muscle damage and soreness as well as fight inflammation and oxidative stress. The anti-inflammatory ingredient has the potential to improve sleep, assist recovery, and promote a runner's ability to train. Tart cherries contain wonderful anti-inflammatory nutrients and taste fantastic. They are an easy addition for simple rehydration or to curb a sweet tooth.

Application:

Consider drinking as much as 10 ounces of tart cherry juice as part of a pre-workout or post-workout regimen. I love the combination of tart cherry juice and Greek yogurt!

Turmeric

Turmeric has many health benefits. Specific to performance, turmeric is a natural anti-inflammatory that can support relieving aches and soreness. Turmeric is a great stand-in for those who are frequently tempted by anti-inflammatory medications for relief from training aches and pains.

Application:

Consider making turmeric tea with warm milk. Add turmeric to meals such as oatmeal, rice and bean-based dishes, eggs, as well as a morning smoothie. There are more therapeutic means to supplement with turmeric or curcumin; however, I recommend incorporating turmeric into a daily fueling regimen through whole foods most often.

Ginger

Ginger contains potent antioxidants with anti-inflammatory properties, such as gingerols. The anti-inflammatory effect supports relief from arthritis and muscle soreness. Ginger is also associated with reducing nausea, upset stomach, and motion sickness.

Application:

Ginger can be included any time of day. Adding ginger to tea and sports drinks is a wonderful way to support a runner's appetite and hydration needs. When shaved into meals, snacks, and sweet treats, ginger roots supports defending against inflammation. Ginger can be used to support an athlete's appetite after a long or hard workout when there is little desire for a recovery snack. Ginger-containing products may also be helpful in soothing an ultra-runner's stomach when faced with nausea and stomach upset during a long event.

Probiotics

Probiotics have immune boosting benefits, but they also support the overall health of any runner, immune-compromised or not. Probiotics support bowel regularity, the absorption of nutrients, the production of vitamins and enzymes, protect gut lining, and more. I recommend whole food probiotics as part of a regular regimen for all runners in support of overall health and performance.

Application:

Probiotics are beneficial any time of day. Choosing from a variety of whole food sources offers the potential for diversity in the probiotic strains consumed and in the gut. Be adventurous in discovering ways to work probiotics into meals and snacks often. Substitute yogurt for sour cream, mayonnaise, cream cheese, and buttermilk. Add sauerkraut to sandwiches, salads, and as a quick snack. Blend plain kefir and fruit for a refreshing smoothie.

Fatty Acids

In regards to a link between the use of fatty acids specific to performance gains, data is limited. On the other hand, there is significant data related to the anti-inflammatory role of beneficial fatty acids in the diet. A deficit in such a powerful anti-inflammatory class of foods could be a contributing factor to an overall systemic inflammatory response. Including food sources of beneficial fatty acids such as oleic acid, omega-3 fatty acids, and alpha linolenic acid supports reducing the inflammatory load on the body.

Application:

Incorporate seeds such as flax and chia into everyday eating through yogurt toppings, breads, and smoothies. Include a fish-based meal a couple days a week. Use avocado as a sandwich spread, pasta sauce, and salad ingredient. Extra virgin olive, high oleic safflower, and avocado oils are great cooking additions.

Supplements

Whole Food First

It is not uncommon to wish a pill could resolve any diet discrepancies. But relying on a pill as a backup has pitfalls. It can create a lax approach to whole food eating and can lead to a watered down diet. Not to mention there is a plethora of nutrients with a whole food approach versus a nutrient isolated supplemental shake or pill.

Supplements may be required to fill gaps. For example, achieving optimal vitamin D can be difficult to achieve during low sunshine months and its limited whole food sources. Another example is a vegan runner who may require B12. Emphasis should always be on whole food first. Any supplementation should be secondary in meeting what a sound whole food diet cannot achieve, not to mask poor eating patterns. Safe, whole food sources do an excellent job of fueling an athlete's needs.

Finding Balance

If supplement use is required, appropriate laboratory testing is the best method to identify how aggressive, if any, supplement use is needed. A full nutrition panel with the Spectracell Micronutrient Test can be a valuable resource to identify insufficiencies in vitamin, mineral, amino acids, fatty acids, as well as assessment of glucose-insulin interaction. Inside Tracker serves as a comprehensive testing resource to assess iron, cortisol, and other inflammatory markers.

To complement any blood work, Cronometer is a useful tool to assess whole food versus supplementation goals, as I referred to in the section on maximizing micronutrients in the "Feed the Immune System" section on page 25. The combination of laboratory testing and optimizing intake of insufficient nutrients through assessment in Cronometer is a complete approach to nutrient assessment and supplement use. Tracking and testing can support any necessary repletion goals as well as excesses in supplement use.

How to Choose a Good Quality Supplement

When you walk into a drug store, grocery store, or supplement center, it is easy to quickly become overwhelmed with supplement options. Supplements are not created equal. It is important to investigate supplements and consider consulting an experienced professional or your physician before choosing any supplement that lines the shelf.

- Seek reputable sources that have good manufacturing practices and certifications, such as certified for sport (NSF).
- A good quality supplement will site research, be involved in conducting research, and often offer education through their website via webinars and educational opportunities. They may be connected with major health organizations in conducting research, such as the Mayo Clinic or Cleveland Clinic.
- Since many herbal supplements do not have third party testing, choose well-known, organic brands of herbal supplements as a safeguard that they have low levels of contamination.
- Aim to choose hypoallergenic supplements. Consider supplements that are free of soy, corn, nuts, and gluten–in addition to any other questionable ingredients that may be problematic specific to how your body responds.
- Single ingredient supplements are more likely to contain the ingredients listed on the label and low in contamination.
- Websites such as Lab Door and Consumer Lab can support weeding out supplements that are not safe, effective, pure, and accurate in what they contain.
- A good supplement will focus on education related to the use of the supplement, not extreme claims. If a supplement sounds too good to be true, it probably is. Avoid any supplements marketed to promote extreme results.

- If a protein powder is deemed appropriate, aim for powders that contain only the protein source as the single ingredient instead of supplements loaded with many hard to understand ingredients. Instead of making a protein drink meal, create a meal using the simple source of protein. This can support homemade protein bars, smoothies using fresh produce, and even to boost a dessert. This allows many great nutrients and antioxidants to enter the meal. In addition, this offers a sense of satisfaction in eating whole food.

Quick Tips:

Caffeine responders, consume a source of caffeine approximately one hour before race start to decrease perceived level of exertion during the race.

- Consume caffeine with carbohydrates after glycogen depleting workouts to support glycogen repletion.
- Overall, limit day-to-day caffeine use, or at least the week leading up to major races, to support a low yet effective race day dose.
- Incorporating beets, beet juice, or beet shots about 1 hour before race start may support performance.
- Include tart cherry juice, turmeric, ginger, and probiotics in everyday eating to take advantage of anti-inflammatory properties.
- Assess micronutrient intake via Cronometer and laboratory testing to assess if supplement use is beneficial.

Choose good quality supplements when necessary for insufficiencies and avoid supplements with overstated claims.

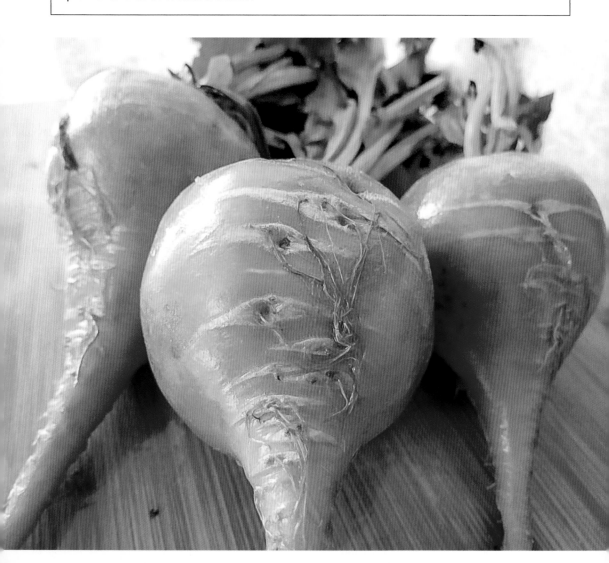

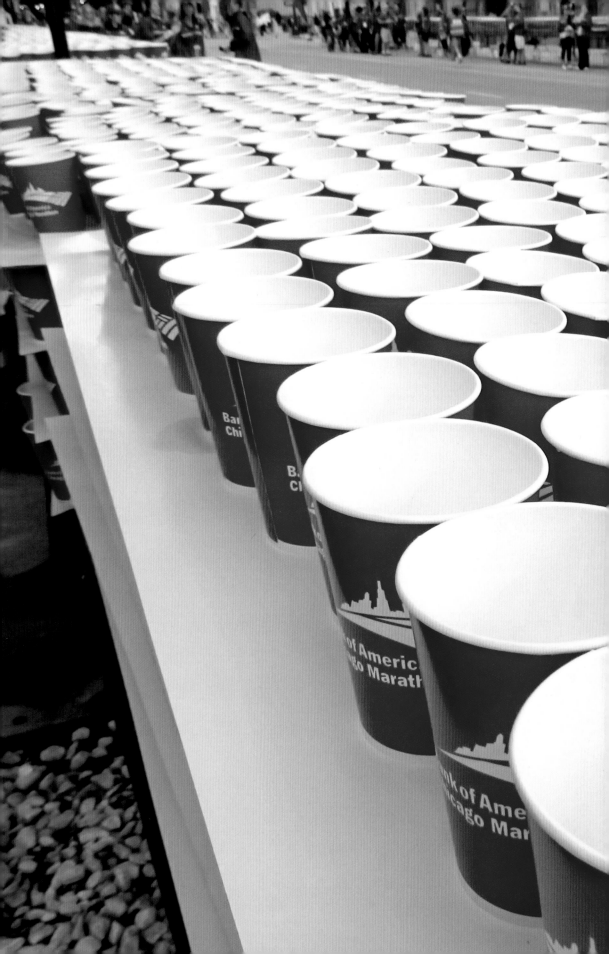

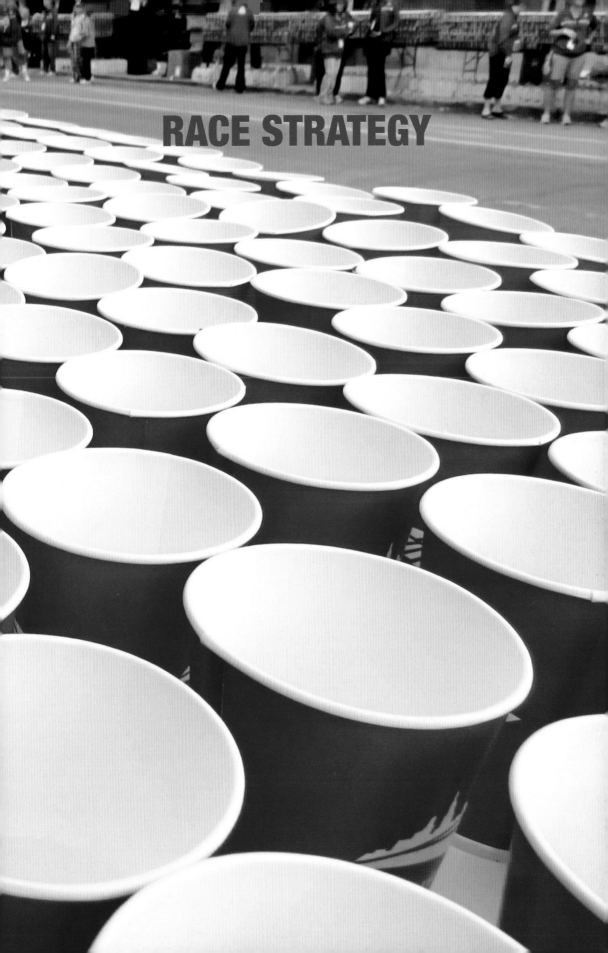

RACE STRATEGY

In preparation for a specific race a runner often considers where they fit in terms of what kind of training regimen to follow. Many training plans described as novice, experienced, and advanced support a specific distance or time goal. Race day nutrition planning is very similar to an overall training strategy.

Just as stages of training involve building upon previous workouts, the same holds true for nutrition concepts. It wouldn't make sense to have a new runner run 20 miles for their first long run. It also wouldn't make sense to tell this same runner to run without taking fuel for long runs, or to take in more fuel than tolerated.

Novice

Nutrition training should emphasize finding palatable, well-tolerated fuel preferences. Test different brands, volumes, and flavors of gel, sports drink, or natural fuel sources during training. The novice should experiment with fueling in order to teach the gut how to take fuel while running, drink to thirst, and develop a system for fueling race day in effort to support a successful finish.

Experienced

Experienced training should hone in on specific nutrition concepts such as breakfast timing and composition; going into a couple shorter runs each week with less fuel; assessing what taking 50 grams of carbohydrate feels like per hour during a long training session versus 30 grams of carbohydrate per hour. The experienced runner should also begin tracking sweat rate trends.

Advanced

The advanced runner is likely targeting a specific time goal with a lot training and has nutrition strategies down pat. This is the time to consider more frequent lab testing, such as regularly tracking ferritin and vitamin D trends. This runner should also be hitting more specific carbohydrate goals in his or her daily food intake, as well as before, during, and after training. He or she may also want to assess enhancements like beet juice as part of a pre-race routine.

Pre-Run Nutrition: Top Tank

This critical meal is for stocking glycogen stores and maintaining optimal blood sugar levels during the initial stages of a race. Eat a carbohydrate-rich meal that includes a source of protein at least 2 to 4 hours before racing. Choose foods to support feeling light, satisfied, and digested. Avoid feeling bogged down by food or hungry during a run. Be sure to test pre-race eating throughout training to determine the best fit.

Where to Begin:

Start with a goal to eat about 40 to 60 grams of carbohydrate with a source of protein for each hour that you eat before a hard workout or race. For example, 1.5 hours before the race eat about 80 grams of carbohydrates and 15 grams of protein. With this meal, drink about 16 to 24 ounces of fluids, aiming for very light-colored urine as a sign of proper hydration. Adapt as tolerated to consuming as much as roughly half your body weight in grams of carbohydrate per hour and the necessary fluid to achieve light-colored urine.

Nutrition During the Run: Practice Makes Perfect

Consuming carbohydrates during long runs will maintain blood glucose and promote carbohydrate oxidation. Fuel the body with a source of carbohydrates for runs lasting 60 to 90 minutes or longer. Both solids and liquids will support performance. Be sure to choose high carbohydrate, low fat, and low fiber foods. The more intense the effort the more likely a runner is to feel sports drink and semi-solid fuel such as gels, honey, and maple syrup are better tolerated and easier to consume.

Dehydration impairs cardiovascular function, temperature regulation, and performance. Consuming adequate fluids will allow a runner to perform at the desired exercise intensity and protect against heat-related injury. Generally speaking, drink to thirst and consume electrolytes with fluids for high sweat loss workouts. Monitoring sweat rate trends in effort to drink according to sweat loss tendencies can support specific fluid and electrolyte goals.

Rule of Thumb:

Aim to consume a minimum of 30 and as much as 90 grams of carbohydrate per hour during exercise lasting greater than 60 to 90 minutes. When carbohydrate intake exceeds about 60 grams of carbohydrate per hour aim for a combination of fructose and glucose fuel sources. Hydrate in effort to maintain within 2 to 3 percent of your starting hydrated body weight as a sign of proper hydration. Weight gain on a run is a sign of taking in too much fluid and should be avoided. Drink electrolyte-containing beverages during high sweat loss workouts with high fluid intake.

Post-Run Nutrition: Master the Mend

Recovery is a key component for successful training and racing for a competitive runner. The more demanding the training load, the more likely a runner will benefit from eating within 30 minutes after long, hard, or intense workouts. Lower mileage or runners seeking weight loss will benefit from timing their next main meal to occur after workouts.

Rule of Thumb:

Consume about 10 to 30 grams of protein and a source of carbohydrate within 30 minutes of training sessions. Strive for half of body weight in grams of carbohydrate as part of the post-workout snack or meal. Eat the next main meal within 1 to 2 hours. Gradually drink in effort to return to pre-run body weight and light-colored urine. Include electrolytes as part of recovery in the form of whole food sources or an electrolyte-containing beverage to support fluid retention.

Advanced Strategy

When to consume carbohydrates relative to training can be somewhat strategic. There is potential in entering some workouts in a somewhat carbohydrate-deprived state to support an efficient fat burning energy system. Most often workouts should be well fueled with carbohydrates to take advantage of optimal performance and fitness gains while reducing stress on the body. In short, a healthy blend between running "low" on carbohydrates and running "high" on carbohydrates can play a role in performance gains.

Most runners can accomplish running "low" or somewhat carbohydrate-deprived by running a couple shorter easy effort early morning runs each week without breakfast. For highly advanced or expert runners I encourage a three-week long-run fueling rotation.

Long Run #1: Perform the run at an easy effort with little to no pre-run or on-the-run carbohydrate-containing fuel. Proper fluids and electrolytes should still be consumed throughout the run. This is ideal for the lowest mileage, most relaxed effort long run of the training cycle.

Long Run #2: Complete the run with half the carbohydrate-containing fuel relative to the ideal race-day fueling routine. This works great when waking up about an hour before a long run to eat half of the typical pre-race breakfast vs. the full breakfast routine. During the run, consume half of the race day carbohydrate fuel routine. For example consume 30 grams of carbohydrate per hour compared to a race day goal of 60 grams of carbohydrate per hour. Proper fluids and electrolytes should still be part of the run. This run can be performed at an easy or moderate effort.

Long Run #3: Perform the full race-day fueling regimen. This works ideal for a goal pace long-run workout or the longest run on the schedule for the three-week rotation. This strategy forces runners to train the gut under race-day conditions. It is very confidence and performance boosting in completing the full race day regimen and knowing what to expect from performance with the full nutrition regimen in place. Strive for optimal fluids, electrolytes, and carbohydrates during the run.

Despite any advanced strategy with occasionally running in a carbohydrate-deprived state, the total daily carbohydrate goal should still be achieved. The runner should return to a carbohydrate-rich diet intake immediately following the run with a carbohydrate-rich post-run meal within 30 minutes of the carbohydrate-deprived effort. In addition, the runner should make up for any potential carbohydrate discrepancies.

Endurance Lover's Carbohydrate Countdown

Carbohydrate intake during the days leading up to a major event shouldn't be too far off from a runner's daily carbohydrate-rich training diet. The trifold combination of rest, typical carbohydrate-rich eating leading up to the race, and sufficient fueling during the race can support a strong finish. However, race nerves, travel, race start time, and lack of knowledge regarding where carbohydrates enter the diet, can make consuming sufficient carbohydrates a bit tricky.

Leading up to a long event like a marathon I like to encourage a three-day carbohydrate-fueling countdown. Maintaining a routine that includes familiar food choices will support typical healthy digestion and regular bowel patterns. If race time is significantly different than the normal running routine, modify training time the week leading up to the race to adjust to the unfamiliar running time.

Three days before the event, a runner should make an effort to consume carbohydrates at all meals and snacks, similar to a typical training day. A low-carbohydrate dinner of spinach salad would therefore shift to a carbohydrate-rich vegetable such as an extra serving of corn or sweet potato.

Two days before the race, begin generally replacing calories from fat sources with carbohydrate calories. For example, instead of buttered bread choose bread with preserves or honey. A dinner meal of rice with six ounces of beef could shift to rice with four ounces lean chicken or fish and carbohydrate-rich black beans. The slow shift should include a target goal to add 50 to 75 grams of carbohydrate versus a typical training day. The runner isn't necessarily eating a whole lot more. There is more so a shift in the calorie sources.

The day before the race would be even more aggressive in shifting fat sources to carbohydrates. Cheese and mayo on a sandwich would be omitted and substituted with fruit, low fat crackers, rice, or a baked potato. A pasta meal would place more emphasis on noodles than a heavy sauce, cheeses, or meat-based toppings.

In addition, consider adding easily digestible, liquid forms of carbohydrates. This can be in the form of juices, milk, or sports drinks. A runner can also add honey to tea or oatmeal. Drinkable carbohydrates and honey or maple syrup can help a runner meet carbohydrate goals without feeling overly full.

The shift in carbohydrates should add another 50 to 75 grams of carbohydrate versus the previous day. The goal is not to feel heavy and bogged down by overeating carbohydrates all day. A runner ideally should frequently snack, never have hunger pangs, and feel comfortably full the day before a race. Limit unfamiliar foods and avoid feeling bloated and heavy from food.

Also, don't fuss too much on race morning if there is a slight gain in weight. The body often holds water when there is an increase in carbohydrate intake. The slightly heavy feeling from holding additional fluids will dissipate early in the race. The morning of the race should be a typical pre-run breakfast routine that has been practiced in training.

Fluid and Electrolytes

The amount of fluid and electrolytes an athlete needs to consume during exercise depends on multiple factors, including environmental conditions, exercise intensity, clothing, nutritional intake, heat acclimation, and fitness level. It is beneficial to know how much sweat is lost during a run in order to better judge how much fluid to ingest. Having a sweat-drenched T-shirt or minimally sweating is not an accurate way to evaluate sweat loss.

A very useful method to assess sweat loss is to weigh oneself before and after exercise. The goal here is finding a balance between how much sweat is lost during exercise with how much fluid and electrolytes is consumed in effort to maintain within 2 to 3 percent of your pre-exercise, hydrated body weight. Sweat rate describes the amount of fluids lost during exercise. Calculating sweat rate is a data-driven way to support hydration confidence and overall performance.

Drinking until thirst is satisfied is an acceptable rule of thumb for an athlete, but tracking general sweat rate patterns only supports supports race-day fueling and confidence. Such information can be very enlightening to a runner who has a history of significantly under- or over-hydrating. It offers the kind of confidence that at the start of any race, under any condition, a race plan can adapt based on previous sweat rate data

Calculate Often

Calculating sweat rate is not a one-time measurement. Because sweat rate changes under variable conditions, it is important to calculate sweat rate under such conditions. A sweat rate taken in the heat of the summer would not be the same as one for a cold December race. By having a general idea of sweat rate trends a runner can adapt to unforeseen weather circumstances based on previous data collected and apply the information that final week leading up to the race.

More is Not Better

Once you've established a sweat rate history, drink slightly less than the calculated rate. It is normal, and even beneficial, to have fluid weight loss during a run. The aim is to maintain fluid weight loss within about 2 to 3 percent of starting, hydrated body weight. Don't feel like you have to see the exact pre-run weight when you weigh immediately after the run. Maintaining within 2 to 3 percent of starting hydrated weight and feeling good throughout the run makes for successful hydration. A runner should never gain weight on a run.

Test Tolerance

A runner may find they sweat at a higher rate than they can tolerate consuming. Take for instance a new runner who calculates a sweat rate of 32 ounces per hour, yet typically drinks only sips in training. This runner is not going to want to apply a 32-ounce per hour race day fluid regimen. Start with comfortable fluid goals and adjust up an ounce or two at a time during training. Test and re-test to determine how much fluid can be comfortably consumed and absorbed while maintaining within about 2 to 3 percent weight loss. A runner with a very high sweat rate is likely to find greater benefit in reducing pace and adapting to conditions versus trying to drink an excessive amount of fluid per hour. High fluid intake should always be paired with an appropriate electrolyte intake, not just consume water alone.

Electrolytes

It is important to achieve a fueling balance of between fluid, carbohydrates, and electrolytes. Drinking only water is likely sufficient for workouts of less than an hour. When a workout exceeds an hour or is high sweat loss, switch to electrolyte-containing beverages.

There are many per hour guidelines for electrolyte consumption goals during exercise. Generally speaking, anywhere from 300 to 1,000 mg of sodium per hour is a very useful guide. However, after working with athletes that consume more salt tablets than they do ounces of fluid, I find myself cautious with per hour sodium recommendations.

Due to many factors that can influence fluid and electrolyte goals, there is no hard-and-fast number for the amount of electrolytes to consume for every runner that toes a starting line. When in doubt, consume electrolytes with fluids versus water alone. The more fluids consumed and the greater the sweat loss, the more electrolytes are needed. Finding the appropriate electrolyte and fluid intake is individual and must be trialed in training, especially if salt tablets are part of a fueling regimen for longer events.

I find pairing sweat rate data with an initial goal of 400 to 600 mg of sodium per liter consumed a nice starting point. Many runners will need to increase this beginning electrolyte range, but I often find runners consuming a 25 mg gel or two with a liter of water per hour during long runs or events like a marathon; or, the opposite in consuming salt tablets and gels, but no fluids. In addition, many runners fail to notice that sport gels and electrolyte tablets can vary significantly in the electrolyte load they carry.

Coupling sweat rate goals with a minimum per liter thought process allows for a healthy initial assessment of electrolyte needs. This should be applied and assessed during shorter training sessions. A runner should adapt as needed based on training assessment for longer training sessions and racing circumstances. A runner may feel well fueled with as much as 250 mg of sodium per 8 ounces, but assessment and building upon the early approach in training is a helpful system to determining individual needs.

A runner who prefers to only consume water with gels during a long event should seek out high electrolyte gels and assess use of electrolyte-only beverages or electrolyte tablets in training. Be aware that drinking only plain water may decrease the desire to actually drink. Electrolyte-containing beverages are pleasing to the palate and encourage the drive to drink.

Sweat Rate How-To
1. Weigh just before exercise begins, while wearing in minimal clothing. This weight should be taken after any eating, drinking, and use of the restroom.

2. Run for approximately one hour, or track total run duration. During this time track the amount of fluid consumed, weather-related conditions, and training intensity. Reattempt sweat rate on a different day if the restroom is needed during the run.

3. Weigh again after the run, while nearly nude. This weight should be taken before any eating, drinking, or use of the restroom.

4. Subtract pre-workout weight from post-workout weight. Multiply the number of pounds lost by 16. Add the number of ounces of fluid consumed during the run (if any) to that number. This number represents ounces. Divide the number of ounces by the duration of the workout, such as one hour. This final number is the number of fluid ounces lost per hour.

5. Track sweat rate trends, conditions, and intensity throughout the season to support hydration judgment and performance.

Sweat Rate Example:
Jon ate a breakfast of ½ c. oatmeal with raisins, a banana, low fat yogurt, 16 ounces of water, and 10 ounces of sports drink 90 minutes before a marathon goal pace workout. One hour before the workout he observed that his urine was still somewhat dark in color. Jon drank another 16 ounces of fluid. About 15 minutes before the goal pace workout Jon drank 6 to 8 ounces of sports drink and used the restroom, noticing light-colored urine. Immediately after drinking and using the restroom, Jon weighed himself in his underwear. His pre-workout weight was 166 pounds. He quickly dressed for the run and began the workout.

During the 90-minute workout Jon drank a combination of water and sports drink for a total of 24 ounces of fluid.

Immediately after the workout Jon weighed himself again in his underwear before drinking any additional fluids or using the restroom. He lost four pounds during the 85-degree workout, weighing in at 162 pounds.

Calculation:

166 pounds −162 pounds = 4 pounds
4 pounds x 16 ounces = 64 ounces
64 ounces + 24 ounces = 88 ounces
88 ounces/1.5 hours exercise = 58.6 ounces per hour sweat rate

Calculation Assessment:

In this example, Jon drank 16 ounces per hour. The information suggests that Jon's sweat rate is about 58 ounces per hour in hot conditions during a high intensity exercise session. Jon's sweat loss percentage was about 2.5 percent of his starting body weight.

The goal is not for Jon to drink 58 ounces of fluid per hour based on this example, but he could progress to and assess drinking closer to 24 to 28 ounces of fluid per hour in effort to maintain just under about 2 percent of his starting body weight for the duration of a full marathon.

After the workout Jon will want to consume fluids and electrolytes in effort to gradually return to his pre-workout, hydrated weight of about 166 pounds; or, Jon can aim for a return of light-colored urine as a sign of rehydration.

Future Training Goal:

Ideally, Jon will want to reassess his sweat rate in the weather conditions expected for race day. If 85-degree weather conditions are expected on marathon day, Jon would want to train his gut to gradually increase to about 25 to 30 ounces per hour during an 85-degree marathon goal pace effort and reassess for maintenance of within roughly a 2 percent loss from his starting, hydrated body weight.

*It's important to note that sweat rate changes related to conditions such as the temperature outside and the intensity of the session. Tracking sweat rates at various times of the year, during different seasons, and at varied training intensities can be a useful tool to support proper hydration.

Salty and Heavy Sweaters

Do you ever notice salt streaks on your clothes or skin? Do your eyes sting from sweat? Do you experience exercise-induced cramps? Do you return from runs with sloshing sounds from your shoes?

If you have answered yes to two or more of these questions then you may belong to the group of athletes often called a "salty sweaters." A salty sweater has a higher than average sodium concentration in his or her sweat. It's important to note that dehydration can also increase the concentration of sodium, as well as potassium, in sweat. There is nothing wrong with being a "salty sweater." As with all athletes, salty sweaters will want to avoid entering a workout thirsty and dehydrated.

Salty sweaters may find consuming an electrolyte-containing beverage to be an essential part of performance. Electrolyte beverages are available in no-calorie, low-calorie, and calorie-containing options. For these salty sweaters, it may be beneficial to consume an electrolyte beverage before high sweat loss workouts. A no-calorie or low-calorie electrolyte beverage is appropriate for heavy sweat loss workouts less than 60 to 90 minutes. Calorie-containing electrolyte beverages are best suited for workouts greater than 60 to 90 minutes. After exercise, aim to replace fluids and electrolytes in effort to return to light-colored urine.

How much are you drinking?

Have you ever questioned how many ounces of fluid you consume during a race or on a run? It's not always easy to look into an aid station cup during a race. Drinking from a water fountain can make exact measurements a challenge.

My favorite trick to help identify how much a runner is drinking is first by measuring one fluid ounce of water. Then, place this ounce of water in your mouth and let it sit there for a few seconds. Feel how much pressure is on the sides of your mouth and the back of your throat. Notice that your mouth feels fairly full. Compare this to what a swallow from the aid station cup is during a race. If forced to compare, is a drink during a race is more like a sip in comparison to the full ounce in the mouth? Maybe each swallow is closer to three-quarters of a mouthful.

Now that you have a better understanding of what an ounce really feels like in the mouth, a runner can better gauge how much you are drinking when measurements aren't available. Compare the swallows during a race to the feeling in your mouth with that ounce of fluid. Count how many full ounces are consumed based on this comparison. At each aid station literally count "one, two, three" until you reach the goal fluid intake in the number of ounces for each aid station. Whether you take half-ounce swallows or choke back a 1.5-ounce mishap, you can better quantify how much is consumed in better meeting your fluid goals.

This is not only a great way to keep track of fluid intake, but it is a pleasant, yet race-ready distraction throughout the race.

Aid Station Success

No matter how experienced the runner, managing aid stations while running a longer race can be tricky. Between dodging fellow runners in combination with gently grasping and tilting back a cup of fluids, while trying to maintain running rhythm, it's enough to deter some runners from taking fluids altogether. Taking fluids while running through an aid station may not always be perfect, but there are strategies to support aid station success.

Take Two: Always take two cups at every aid station. Even if a runner feels they only need one cup, take two. Since a runner does not know what to expect in the cup it only makes sense to have a second cup as a backup.

Pinch one cup completely shut while drinking from the other to minimize spilling and preserve the second cup of fluids if it is needed. This strategy is also a great way to be prepared if too much of the essential fluids spill from the first cup, or if a single cup only contains 1 to 2 ounces and will fall short meeting fluid goals.

The Egg: While approaching the aid station, think of the cup as a delicate egg. Grabbing the cup too firmly it will "break" the egg and spill all over. This fairly gentle, yet firm, grab is a great mental approach to a successful fluid-filled grab.

The Pinch: Gently pinching half of the cup shut before drinking helps to minimize water or sports drink splashing back in the eyes. The ideal pinch method becomes a matter of personal preference.

Practice Makes Perfect: The more often a runner takes fluids from a race, the more comfortable he or she becomes with taking aid station fluids. Fluency with the aid station is another way to become "race fit."

   If the opportunity to race often is limited, practicing at home works great. Line a few fluid-filled Dixie cups on the roof or hood of a car to develop aid station confidence. Pretend the car is lined with an awesome staff of aid station volunteers and practice grabbing a Dixie cup "egg" with each pass.

The Mill: Workouts performed on a treadmill are another great way to practice fueling while running. Be it drinking from a water bottle as an elite at 5:30 pace or simply learning how to time breathing rhythm with holding fluids in the mouth, foot plant, and swallow. Consider scheduling a nutrition treadmill workout with planned race day fuel within arm's reach for practicing race day nutrition.

Quick Tips:
As a starting point, begin by consuming 40 to 60 grams of carbohydrate for each hour that you eat before a workout or race. Build as tolerated to eating about half of body weight in grams of carbohydrate with a source of protein per hour.

- During competition, eat at least 30 and as much as 90 grams of carbohydrate per hour for workouts lasting greater than 60 to 90 minutes.
- After demanding workouts and races, aim to eat about half of your body weight in grams of carbohydrate and 10 to 30 grams of protein within 30 minutes.
- Low-mileage or runners seeking weight loss should eat their next main meal soon after demanding workouts or races.
- Light-colored urine is a sign of proper hydration before, during, and after workouts.
- Dark-colored urine is a sign of poor hydration throughout the day as well as before, during, and after workouts.
- Learn how to calculate sweat rate and track sweat rate trends in various conditions to gain a better understanding of individual fluid needs.
- Drink according to sweat rate during exercise in effort to maintain within 2 to 3 percent of your hydrated, pre-exercise weight.
- Gaining weight during a workout is a sign of drinking too much fluid and/or insufficient electrolytes during the workout.
- Practice proper hydration during training sessions to support performance and train the gut to better tolerate fluid goals.

- Break fluid consumption up over the course of the hour versus drinking 20 ounces in a single stop.
- Strive to consume fuel at frequent steady intervals throughout a run.
- Practice aid station success during training to become more comfortable with race day circumstances.

Proper Hydration is a Critical Determinant in the Body's Ability to Train, Compete, and Recover Successfully

Before Exercise

- Start exercise hydrated by drinking throughout the day.
- Slowly drink fluids in aiming for light-colored urine.
- Consume electrolyte-containing beverages or foods to stimulate thirst and retain fluids.

During Exercise

- Sweat loss and hydration needs vary among athletes.
- Listen to your body and drink with signs of thirst.
- Monitor sweat loss before and after exercise using body weight changes in effort to maintain within 2–3 percent of your starting, hydrated body weight.
- Avoid drinking more fluid than is needed to replace sweat loss.
- Avoid gaining weight, a sign of taking in too much fluid.
- Include a source of electrolytes during high sweat loss workouts.
- During workouts greater than 60–90 minutes, include carbohydrates for energy and electrolytes to retain hydration and stimulate thirst.
- Environment such as temperature, sun exposure, protective clothing, and humidity influence the amount of sweat produced during exercise.

After Exercise

- Aim to gradually consume fluid at a steady rate in effort to return to pre-run hydrated body weight
- Look for a return to light-colored urine.
- Consume sodium-containing beverages, light snacks, or the next main meal to help retain fluids and stimulate thirst.

—Support Daily Hydration—

* Start the day by drinking 16–20 swallows of water first thing in the morning.

* Consume 16–20 swallows of water with meals and snacks.

* Before drinking soda, coffee, and other forms of energy beverages drink 16–20 swallows of water.

* Aim for light-colored urine as an indicator of proper hydration throughout the day.

* Keep a refillable water bottle on hand for easy access and frequent fluid refills.

*Food sources such as fruit, vegetables, broth soups, and smoothies support hydration.

Olympic Marathon Trials 2012 Race Day Example

In an effort to support the race day thought process, I thought I would share my marathon stats from the 2012 Olympic Team Trials Marathon. The word "stats" might imply splits, distances, and personal bests. My marathon stats involve carbohydrates, calories, and ounces—how I fueled before, during, and after the marathon. These exact numbers won't necessarily work for everyone. My fueling plan was based on my sweat rate, personal experience, and application of evidence-based information.

Before the Race:

Within the final 2.5 hours leading up to race start I consumed:

> 1 large cinnamon raisin bagel
> A medium banana
> Roughly 14 ounces high electrolyte sports drink
> 1 cup of strong coffee
> Roughly 25 to 30 ounces of water

Energy Consumed: 115 g carb, 735 mg sodium, 11 g protein, and 525 calories

Energy Burned: 10-minute run/warm up (approx.100 calories burned)

During the Race

The race day temperature ended up being cooler than previously expected. As a result I dropped my fluid consumption goal based on sweat rate trends that had been calculated at similar temperatures in training. The race day temperature placed my sweat rate at about 24 to 25 ounces per hour. Since it is normal and even a slight advantage to lose a small percentage of weight during the race, I dropped my fluid goals to about 20 to 22 ounces per hour.

I had 8 ounces of fluid in all of the nine bottles available for the elite athletes. Six of the bottles contained high electrolyte sports drink and the other three bottles contained water to take with high electrolyte gel. I took about 6–7 ounces from most of the sports drink–filled bottles at miles 3.2, 6, 11.2, 14, and 19.2 miles. At miles 8.6 and 16.6, I took a whole gel with about 8 ounces of water. At mile 22 I took closer to half a gel with about 7 to 8 ounces of water. For the final fluid station at 24.6, I took about 4 ounces of sports drink.

During the 2 hours and 48 minute duration of the race I consumed:

> Roughly 57–60 ounces of fluid = 20–21 ounces/hour

Roughly 143 g carbohydrate = 50–52 grams of carbohydrate/hour
Roughly 1,310 mg sodium = 720–760 mg sodium/liter fluids consumed and
462 mg sodium per hour

Energy Consumed: about 564 calories

Energy Burned: As per my Garmin watch, about 2,571 calories

After the Race (within 30 minutes):

I casually drank almost a bottle and a half of water and a pre-packed recovery bar.

Energy Consumed: 250 calories, 43 carbohydrates, 140 mg sodium, 10 grams of protein, and 25 to 30 ounces of water

The Grand Total by 11:15 a.m.:

Energy Consumed: 306 grams of carbohydrate, 1,339 calories

Energy Burned: about 2,700 calories burned with running alone

That's a lot of fuel!
I never felt faded during the race. I ran exactly in the time range that was expected based on my fitness going into the race with a 2:48:29 finish time. I felt no reflection of dwindling energy; and in fact, over the last 4 miles I passed about fifteen women and felt great. This makes for the best kind of marathon experience—owning the last 6 miles versus conceding to them.

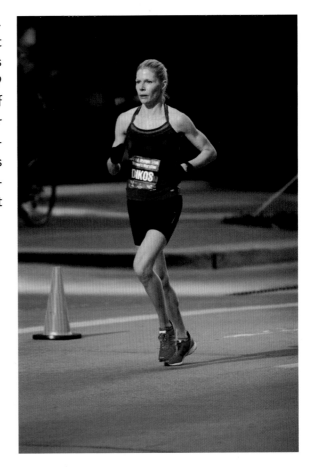

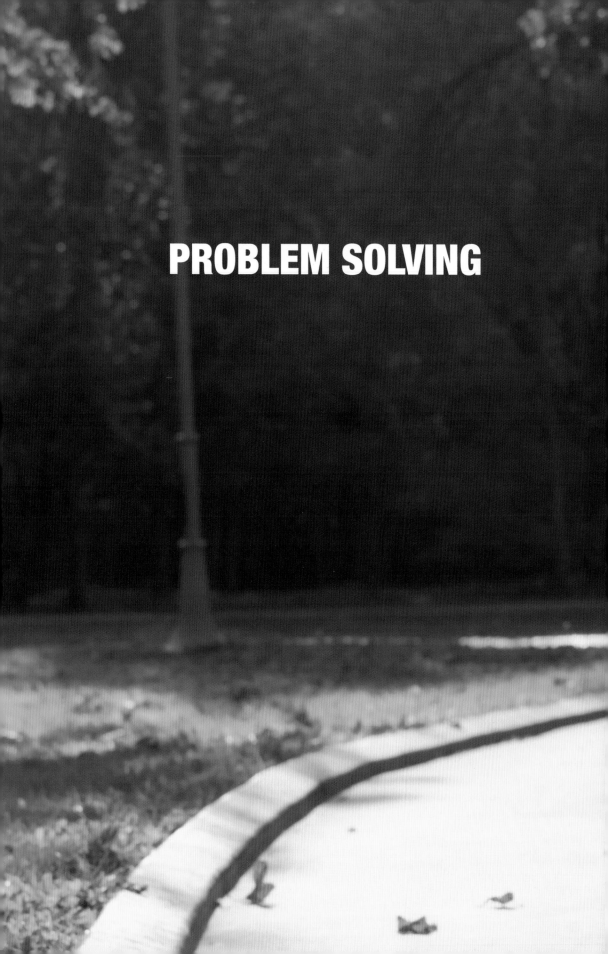

PROBLEM SOLVING

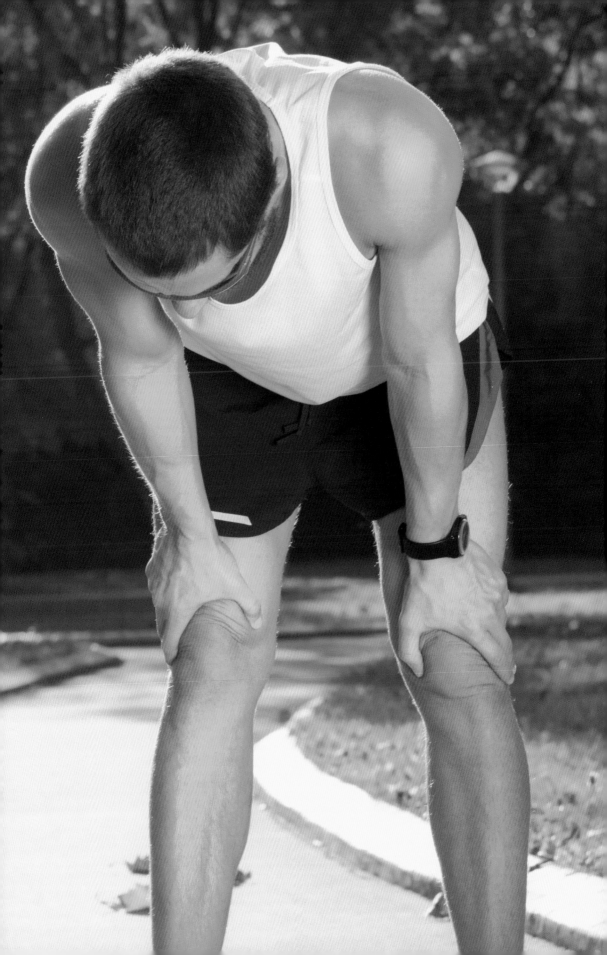

Time Crunch: Finding the Time to Cook

As an athlete, it is instinctive to push limits. It's not uncommon to start the day with a 5 a.m. run in an effort to maintain health, optimize performance, and fit all of the necessary tasks into the day. Many sacrifices come with pushing these limits, and without necessarily knowing it, proper nutrition is often forfeited.

An extra 15 minutes added to a workout may be the difference between a 4-mile run and a 6-mile run. For many runners pursuing convenient food sources is worth every last minute and mile. Are the extra 15 minutes worth skipping a quality meal, reaching for a sports performance bar, or conceding to trying the latest protein shake on the market?

Great fueling can still be convenient. Plan ahead by making extra portions at meals as often as possible. Instead of boiling two eggs for a meal, boil six, and store the extras in the refrigerator for an easy go-to protein to complement a carbohydrate-rich snack.

Explore the freezer section of the grocery store. Bypass prepackaged, full-meal products available in a bag or box. Stick with simple frozen ingredients that can be heated and paired with any combination of fresh ingredients from the refrigerator. A great savory vegetable sauté can be paired with a plain frozen brown rice, and extra boiled eggs from the previous day for a quick and easy meal.

Freeze any prepared foods when there is an opportunity for extra food prep. Pancakes and spelt pitas are delicious toasted from the freezer. Chop fresh vegetables and store them in the freezer to limit chopping time for rushed meals.

When in doubt remember, food doesn't have to be complicated. A healthy diet can be achieved without meals that require hours of food prep and cooking. Don't feel bound to the thinking that meals are either a deluxe dinner or fast food. Let's be practical. There will always be days the mere thought of cooking is fatiguing and it's hard to know where to even begin. Choose simple, fresh ingredients and make the most of what is available.

Dining Out and Lacing Up

After months of preparation, traveling to a race facing many food unknowns can be anxiety inducing. The idea that the wrong meal may mean a bathroom stop in the midst of a personal record performance is heartbreaking. When in doubt, stick with familiar foods as often as possible. Travel with or visit a grocery store for a supply of fresh fruit, crackers, rice cakes, and other comfortable food choices that can fill any gaps that a less than ideal dining out experience is missing. Choose from "fit-friendly" menu items as often as possible to support race day success.

"Fit-Friendly" Menu Items

- Baked sweet potato (limit bacon, butter, cheese, and sour cream)

- Bison
- Bran muffin or cereal
- Broth, bean, or lentil based soups
- Chicken, grilled or broiled
- Chili cup
- Deli sandwich on whole grain
- Edamame
- Egg, egg white, egg substitute omelets with vegetables and lean proteins
- Fish–grilled or baked tilapia, salmon, cod, shrimp, and scallops
- Fish tacos in soft shell-grilled tilapia, cod, salmon, shrimp
- Flatbread or whole grain crust pizza (limit cheese and fatty meat toppings)
- Fresh fruit
- Mussels
- Oatmeal
- Potatoes, white or sweet
- Quinoa
- Rice–preferably steamed brown rice or wild rice
- Seared tuna
- Steamed and sautéed vegetables
- Steak–sirloin or round
- Turkey–grilled or broiled
- Whole Grain–breads, pasta, tortilla, cereals, crackers, wraps, buns, and crust

Heavy Meal Red Flags

Some menu items carry a deceivingly significant fat and calorie load. Such options should be avoided or significantly portion controlled if they are part of a pre-race regimen. Red flag foods are more likely to contribute to gastrointestinal distress; or, they are less likely to offer the ratio of pre-race macronutrients to support great racing.

- Artichoke dip
- Battered fish
- Biscuits and gravy
- Buffalo wings
- Burgers–prepared extra thick on buttered buns and loaded with fried onions, and heavy with mayonnaise sauces
- Chicken, tuna, crab, and pasta salads made with heavy mayonnaise
- Cream soup, such as broccoli and cheese, chowder, bisque, and loaded potato
- Creamy pastas such as macaroni and cheese, Alfredo, and Carbonara
- Creamed spinach
- French fries, fried potatoes, waffle fries, fried potato slices
- Fried chicken or pork
- Fried Rice

- Hash browns
- Omelets –when made with three to five whole eggs, stuffed with fatty meats, excessive cheese, and covered with creamy sauces
- Ribs
- Steak, rib eye, T-bone, New York strip, porterhouse

Restaurant Terms to Avoid or Practice Portion Control

Aioli	Hollandaise
Au gratin	Loaded
Battered	Pan-fried
Bottomless	Refried
Bisque	Roux
Breaded	Scalloped
Crispy	Scampi
Crunchy	Stuffed
Casserole	Smothered
Country-style	Tempura
Deep-fried	Value
Fritters	White sauce
Golden	

Poor Recovery

Have you ever felt a lack of "pop" during a workout? It's not a feeling of not being able to finish, or just feeling plain bad. It's a sense that no matter how hard the body is pushed it just won't reach the flying sensation that comes with a great workout. There are a number of factors that contribute to the disappointing run.

Eating soon after a workout will support, strengthen, and protect the body's ability to adapt to training and demand more out of training. Effective refueling should include protein to support muscle repair and synthesis, carbohydrates to replenish the body's carbohydrate (glycogen) energy stores and sustain high intensity training, as well as fluid and electrolytes to replace sweat loss. Eating such food sources within 30 minutes after a demanding training session maximizes today's workout and energizes tomorrow's workout.

While every run won't be perfect, the ultimate goal of recovery nutrition is to facilitate returning the body to a "normal" state as to continue high intensity training with as little interruption as possible. Specific nutrition recovery goals should be tailored based on training, body size and composition, performance goals, as well as the stress level of the runner. Recovery nutrition should be applied soon after taxing workouts. Interpretation of a taxing workout varies from runner to runner.

Carbohydrates

Carbohydrate intake is a "slow to recover" factor. Low carbohydrate eating can leave the body deprived of valuable energy and induce stress for a training runner. Since glucose is the body's primary source of energy, stored in the form of glycogen from carbohydrates, it doesn't make sense for a runner to deny such a valuable fuel source day-after-day.

It's important for an athlete to keep a running tally, even if just a general assessment, of how many grams of carbohydrate are consumed in the average day. Compare the numbers to what should be consumed based on your body weight, as described on page 13. If there is a big discrepancy between the two, restructuring of the diet is likely necessary. Aim to slowly build over time to your ideal carbohydrate range.

If general daily carbohydrate intake is sufficient, consider timing. Optimize the window before and after training. For example, if fuel is skipped after most runs, aim to train the gut to get used to eating within 15 to 30 minutes of training sessions. Carbohydrates with a source of protein should be paired together. If a post-run "protein" shake is the standard recovery practice, yet it contains only 10 grams of carbohydrate, be sure to restructure the meal with carbohydrates as the main fuel and paired with a source of protein.

Recovery nutrition doesn't necessarily mean adding snacks or calories to the day. A runner seeking weight loss would benefit from scheduling workouts to occur just before the next main meal, such as prior to breakfast, lunch, or dinner, as to not add a significant calorie load while supporting recovery and weight management goals.

Fight Inflammation with Food

The body is constantly defending against unwanted inflammation, especially when pushing physical limitations. There was a time when I thought I needed to defend against inflammation and injury by resorting to too much over-the-counter anti-inflammatory use. Without the emotional, blinded, do-or-die spirit I had at the time, I now look back and realize I was likely resorting to anti-inflammatories as a means to run through more inflammation than I should have been.

The end result was sub-par performances and a hard-to-recover-from injury. The possibility of a quick reduction in inflammation muddled my judgment of a true need for rest. There are many benefits to listening to the body and incorporating natural anti-inflammatories as well as rest days or rest cycles in training. After a long, hard road back to feeling normal again I decided to switch my mentality and seek natural ways to fight inflammation on a more regular basis.

By fighting inflammation with food there is a greater understanding for what the body is trying to communicate. Inflammation fighting foods are rich in antioxidants, minerals, and essential fatty acids.

Great sources include:

- Green leafy vegetables, broccoli, bell peppers, pineapple, citrus, berries, seafood, nuts, seeds, beans, lentils, avocado, olive, mushrooms, whole grains, sweet potato, banana, and grass-fed meat and dairy.

Quick Tips:
- To support recovery, pair carbohydrates with protein within 30 minutes of hard, long, or taxing efforts, consuming about half of body weigh in grams of carbohydrate and 10 to 30 grams of protein.
- Ensure fluids and electrolytes are part of recovery fueling and recognize if it takes several hours to urinate for the first time after workouts.
- Fight inflammation with foods rich in antioxidants, minerals, and essential fatty acids.

Runner Cravings

There are three main cravings runners want most often:

1. Chocolate
2. Prepackaged salty foods such as chips, crackers, and pretzels
3. Sweets such as cookies, candy, and sugar beverages

Cravings can become so intense that the diet dominates with empty food sources in effort to suppress the powerful urge to indulge. Such cravings may be the body communicating something deeper than a desire to enjoy a savory piece of chocolate.

Identify Your Triggers

Sweets

- Going too long without eating can cause low blood sugar and a craving for quick carbohydrates. Plan ahead with regular meals and snacks.
- A diet insufficient in carbohydrates causes the body to produce a hormone that sends a message to eat more carbohydrates. This contributes to a craving for sweets as a source of quick carbohydrates. Consider increasing quality carbohydrate sources such as brown rice, bread, oatmeal, bran cereal, sweet potatoes, fruit, quinoa, and whole grain pasta.

- A lack of sleep interferes with the balance of hormones that regulate hunger and feeling satisfied. In response the body may seek a quick energy source in the form of sweets and refined sugars. Be sure to get sufficient sleep and take naps as needed.
- Anemia or low iron can cause fatigue, which contributes to an increased craving for quick energy sources and refined sugars. Incorporate iron-rich foods such as beef, chicken, quinoa, clams, oysters, mussels, green leafy vegetables, beans, lentils, pumpkin seeds, and fortified cereals.
- Lack of balance in consuming protein, carbohydrates, and fat at meals and snacks can interfere with blood sugar levels and hormones. Find the right balance of carbohydrates, protein, and fat at meals and snacks.
- Eating too many processed, low fiber carbohydrates can cause a quick spike in blood sugar followed by a quick drop, stimulating hunger and carbohydrate cravings. Choose high quality carbohydrates most often.

Chocolate

- Insufficient magnesium can contribute to a craving for chocolate as dark chocolate is a source of magnesium. Increase magnesium-rich foods such as green leafy vegetables, bran cereals, nuts, seeds, fish, avocado, and bananas.
- Low fat or an imbalance of healthy fat in the form of oleic and omega-3 fatty acids can trigger the urge to reach for chocolate. Incorporate more olive oil, high oleic safflower oil, avocado, walnuts, fatty fish, chia and flax seed into everyday eating.

Salty Foods

- A desire for prepackaged salty foods may be a sign of general dehydration from day-to-day activity. First, assess if a simple glass or two of water kills the desire to snack on salty chips. If that doesn't do the trick, consider adjusting food choices. A broth-based soup rich in quality ingredients will support rehydration, recovery, and offer an array of nutrients while hydrating. Include natural sodium-rich foods such as cottage cheese and celery.
- Electrolytes lost from a high sweat loss workout need to be replaced. Consider an electrolyte replacement drink during workouts and include electrolyte-rich food choices as part of recovery. Add a touch of extra high quality salt to quality whole food choices. For example, sprinkle a touch of salt on a baked sweet potato; or top a sweet potato with a sodium rich protein source such as a cup of chili.

Top Tips to Eating Your Way out of a Sweet Tooth

1. Avoid going long windows of time without eating.
2. Increase intake of quality carbohydrate sources at each meal and snack.
3. Reach for fruit first. Maintain a goal of eating two to five pieces of fruit a day.
4. Choose fiber-rich carbohydrates most often.

Easy Sweet Treats for Runners

- Smoothies: Combine ingredients like fruit, yogurt, milk, nuts or nut butters, avocado, and green leafy vegetables.
- Dark Chocolate: Pair 65 percent or greater cocoa dark chocolate with a few walnuts and raisins.
- Greek yogurt: Add options such as fresh fruit, seeds, nuts, cocoa powder, and granola.
- Fresh fruit, cooked fruit, and fruit-based popsicles.
- Frozen ripe banana chunks.
- Hot chocolate made with milk or chocolate milk.
- Avocado-based pudding.

Sweet Substitutions: *Aim for sweets with nutrient-rich ingredients.*

White Flour: Prepare the recipe with whole grain flour for at least half of what the recipe calls for in white flour. Great substitutions to rotate include oat, wheat, brown rice, spelt, buckwheat, and teff. Look for whole grain flours in the list of ingredients as the first or second ingredient.

Sugar: Consider decreasing the amount of sugar in a recipe or use forms of sugar that carry health benefits such as dates and other dried or fresh fruit, pure maple syrup, molasses, fruit purees, and local honey.

Fats: Modify recipes using a rotation of nutrient dense, high quality fats such as olive oil, high oleic safflower oil, nuts, avocado, grass-fed butter, and seeds. Seek good quality fats on ingredient labels.

Fruit: Choose recipes rich in fresh or dried fruit.

Fueling a Nervous Appetite

The hours leading up to a race can really kill a hearty, heavy training appetite. Proper fueling is required the final hours in topping glycogen stores and aiding a strong performance.

- Choose moist, easy to swallow ingredients. A dry bagel may not go down as well as a bagel topped with yogurt, banana, and honey.
- Drinkable fuel sources such as juice, milks, sports drink, and kefir are easy to swallow, hydrating, and offer a source of carbohydrates.
- For an early morning race, wake with plenty of time for a slow to consume meal and mentally prepare for the race. Rushing to prepare can make a nervous meal get brushed to the side.

Lack of Menstruation

An initial factor a female runner needs to consider with a lack of menstruation is to ensure sufficient calories are consumed daily. A runner with a history of insufficient overall calorie intake should begin with effort to consume 250 or more calories daily until menses resumes. The longer a runner has gone without a menstrual cycle related to inadequate calorie intake, the longer it will likely take for menses to return.

When looking for a solution, consider the evaluation of micronutrients such as zinc, magnesium, chromium, and iron disorders such as iron-overload seen with hemochromatosis. Addressing insufficiencies and excesses may support return of menses. Testing for chronically elevated cortisol levels may be another means to assess stress load for the female runner. Strategies such as increasing carbohydrates and sleep while reducing training load may support healthy cortisol response and menstrual function.

Bone Health

Proper training, shoes, genetics, hormones, and nutrition all factor in to bone health. A high rate of stress fractures may be indicating a high dietary stress load on the body. A synergy of nutrients such as calcium, vitamin D, magnesium, vitamin K, and zinc all play a role in bone health.

A great starting point for the runner suffering frequent fractures is laboratory evaluation of vitamin D status. Not only does a low vitamin play a major role in bone health, low vitamin D can trigger chronic inflammation and immune response. Supplementation of vitamin D3 may be required at least through low sun exposure months.

As with the female runner lacking menstruation, chronically elevated cortisol and overtraining plays a role in bone health. Effort should be made to increase carbohydrate intake and sleep while reducing training load to support healthy cortisol response and bone health.

Gastrointestinal Distress

There are a number of reasons why a runner may experience gastrointestinal distress. Lactose intolerance, an imbalance of healthy bacteria in the gut, more effort toward "training the gut" to tolerate fuel before or during exercise, timing of fiber intake, high fat intake, dehydration, and use of NSAIDS are just some of the potential contributing factors.

Dairy

Runners who experience gastrointestinal distress related to dairy products may need to avoid dairy in the race-day meal planning. Dairy may need to be eliminated the day before a race as well. Consider dairy alternatives such as almond, cashew, soy, flax, and coconut milks and yogurts.

A runner who may be experiencing lactose intolerance may find they tolerate yogurts, kefir, and even some cheeses just fine. Through a process of elimination and slowly adding one food back at a time, try to determine which dairy sources will be the best fit.

Keep in mind that the nutrition content of most non-dairy products will not be an equal trade for dairy sources. The protein content is often much less and fat content may be much greater. This is not a problem as long as appropriate adjustments and replacements are made in meeting a healthy macronutrient balance of the meal or snack.

Probiotics

Those who suffer from gastrointestinal distress may want to explore increasing probiotic-rich foods sources, and possibly supplementation to support symptom relief. Begin by gradually including more yogurt, kefir, sauerkraut, kombucha, and kimchi. If a significant increase in bloating occurs, reduce the amount consumed and gradually rebuild as tolerated.

An increase in bloating, a mild rash, bowel changes (diarrhea or constipation), early signs of a cold, and other similar mild symptoms may occur related to healthy changes of gut bacteria. Most often, probiotic symptoms should be mild. The aim is to never create significant distress.

Lactobacillus and bifidobacterium strains are most researched for efficacy. Research and discuss with your doctor or healthcare professional the best probiotic strain to pair well with the symptoms experienced. If a runner is immunocompromised, a high dose probiotic regimen may stir up an unsafe inflammatory response.

Pairing Fluid with Solids

During longer training sessions and events such as the marathon, consuming carbohydrates during the run spares glycogen and supports performance. When consuming fuel it is important to consider the type of fuel and the combination of sources. Most often runners will want to avoid combining sports drink with other carbohydrate-rich fuel sources, such as gels, sport chews, and beans, at the same time.

Fuel sources should be broken up over the course of each hour to avoid the risk of creating an environment in the gut that is too concentrated. Consume gels, honey sandwiches, maple syrup, sport chews, beans, and other similar forms of fuel with water or an electrolyte-only beverage. Wait about 10 to 15 minutes, and then consume a sports drink only. Create a rotation every 10 to 15 minutes between fuel sources.

Be sure to take solid forms of fuel with 4 to 8 ounces of water or an electrolyte-only beverage. Consuming the solid forms of fuel without sufficient fluids can induce gastrointestinal distress and possibly a bathroom stop.

Healthy Elimination

Most experienced runners would agree that a run feels lighter and more successful with healthy elimination before the run. It also reduces the risk of gastrointestinal upset on the run. Healthy elimination is an important part of pre-race strategy and overall health.

Healthy elimination begins with a healthy intake of fiber and fluids. Runners should be consuming at least 25 to 35 grams of fiber daily. Fiber paired with sufficient fluids is essential. Be sure to drink the sixteen to twenty swallows of fluids at meals and snacks and avoid dehydration.

An early morning runner will want to wake with enough time to allow the body to adjust from sleep to wake. A rushed and anxious runner can lead to a constipated runner. Consider sipping a warm beverage such as tea, coffee, juice, or milk to get the bowels moving. A beverage that contains caffeine can also support elimination.

It is not uncommon for a runner with high-energy demands, and therefore a high volume of food intake, to eliminate more than once a day. However, experiencing frequent loose or liquid bowel movements may suggest further investigation is warranted. Evaluate overall fiber intake for excesses and the ratio of sources between soluble versus insoluble fiber. Consider laboratory evaluation and discussion with a health care professional about gut-supporting nutrients such as zinc, L-glutamine, sodium butyrate, and probiotics.

Weight Management

Loss

The macronutrient goal for a runner looking to lose weight begins by targeting the low end of the macronutrient range for fat and carbohydrates and upper end of protein based on body weight and training. Adjustments to the macronutrient goal would be made based on rate of loss with a goal to lose no more than one to two pounds per week. Weight loss that is too rapid can lead to hard to control cravings, increase in stress and injury, or rebound weight gain.

If tracking macronutrients does not meet quality of life objectives with desired weight loss, consider some of the following weight loss tips:

- Leave each meal or snack wanting to take three more bites. If after 20 to 30 minutes true hunger cues remain, have a few more bites. Slow eating down in such a way that allows the brain enough time to reconigize sufficient fuel was consumed at the meal.
- Go to bed feeling tempted to have a snack. This does not mean you have to go to bed with a intense hunger. Late night overeating is a frequent occurance among athletes that can become excess. The aim is to go to bed feeling somewhat light.
- Limit mindless snacking. Define the meals and snacks for eating. Outside of these windows, avoid walking past the pantry, candy bowl, or snack station and munching all day long.
- Stay hydrated. Runners often confuse hunger cues with thirst cues. Biting into a juicy apple can offer a hydrating sense of satisfaction that can be confused with fulfilling a hunger, as does replacing electrolytes with salty chips. First drink a tall glass of water or an electrolyte-only beverage. After about 10 to 15 minutes, reassess if true hunger remains.
- Serve meals from the stovetop. When food is centered at the table it is easy to keep munching on the meal despite feeling satisfied.
- Remove wet clothing soon after a run and put on dry clothing before eating. The post-run snack can become excessive if the body remains chilled in wet running clothes.
- Assess stress load. Holding extra weight may be related to a high stress load and elevated cortisol. Ensure sufficient rest cycles, sleep, carbohydrates, and amino acids are part of training.

Gain

Maintaining or gaining weight can be just as difficult for some athletes as it is for others to lose. Avoid going too long without eating. Eat often enough that the body never truly gets the opportunity to experience hunger pangs. If the diet is very high in fiber, reducing the fiber load may be less filling and leave room for sufficient calories.

A runner struggling to maintain weight will find drinkable calories a big help in meeting calorie needs without feeling overly full. Great options include fruit and vegetable juices, milk, chocolate milk, smoothies, kefir, and coconut water. Consume drinkable calories at meals as well as for general daily hydration.

Sneaking in calories as often as possible may be needed. One way to accomplish this is through healthy fats. Apply a layer of flax oil to toast before topping it with sandwich toppings or fruit preserves; add flax, olive, or avocado oil to smoothies and oatmeal; roast vegetables with an extra tablespoon of the healthy oils.

While healthy fats are helpful to adding calories, it is important to attain sufficient carbohydrates. Choose dense breads and cereals. Concentrated carbohydrate sources like dried fruit, honey, and maple syrup may support the extra boost to meals and snacks needed to maintain weight. Consider a bowl of fresh fruit topped with yogurt, honey, dried fruit, and granola tossed in flax oil. The snack can be made quite dense for low volume eating.

Blend ingredients to reduce the volume when necessary. Blended or mashed sweet potato can work well in a homemade spaghetti sauce, soup, or chili. Blend an avocado into a smoothie. Mash or blend black or garbanzo beans and combine with olive oil and tahini to make a dense dip.

Anemia

A runner with anemia is likely to experience increasing fatigue, weakness, and lack of stamina. It certainly can affect running, but also slowly creeps into other aspects of active life with a shortness of breath, headaches, difficulty concentrating, irritability, dizziness and a rapid heartbeat with small tasks like climbing stairs or carrying groceries.

Iron is essential for oxygen transport. When deficient, oxygen cannot be carried to tissue and working muscles leading to fatigue, deterioration in performance, and even a decline in healthy immune function. Iron deficiency without anemia is a condition in which hemoglobin levels are normal, but serum ferritin is reduced.

Endurance athletes should consider screening not only for anemia but also for low ferritin. Serum ferritin is not a lab always checked by a medical practitioner.

A runner with normal iron status will not feel any enhancement in performance with supplementation. However athletes with normal iron status who attempt to increase red blood cells, such as training at altitude, may benefit from iron supplementation. Runners should follow through with a proper anemia and iron workup before supplementation. Iron-overload is a condition that can be very dangerous.

If iron status is in question, making effort to increase iron through whole food is a great start.

- Eat iron-fortified grain products and cereals. Keep in mind not all cereals are fortified and may contain poor quality ingredients. Quality cereals such as fortified bran flakes not only serve as a great recovery snack, but can also function as a source of iron.

- Include dark leafy greens as often as you can. A 1/2 c. serving of cooked spinach offers about 3.2 mg of iron. Dark green leafy vegetables can make a delicious salad or simply sneak them into dishes such as rice, spaghetti sauce, or even a chili.
- A well-known source of iron is red meat. A 3-ounce serving provides about 3.2 mg of iron. Enjoy a serving of lean red meat several times a week to take advantage of its iron content.
- Beans and lentils are an easy topping or meal. Include beans with pasta dishes, top them on salad, or bake them for a nice nutty crunch.
- A less obvious source of iron is blackstrap molasses. Eating 1 tablespoon of black strap molasses offers about 20 percent of the daily value of iron. Incorporate molasses into cooking dishes like mashed sweet potatoes, pancakes, squash, and baked beans.
- Pair iron-rich food sources with vitamin C rich food sources to support iron absorption.
- Limit consuming iron-rich food sources with calcium-rich food sources since calcium inhibits iron absorption.

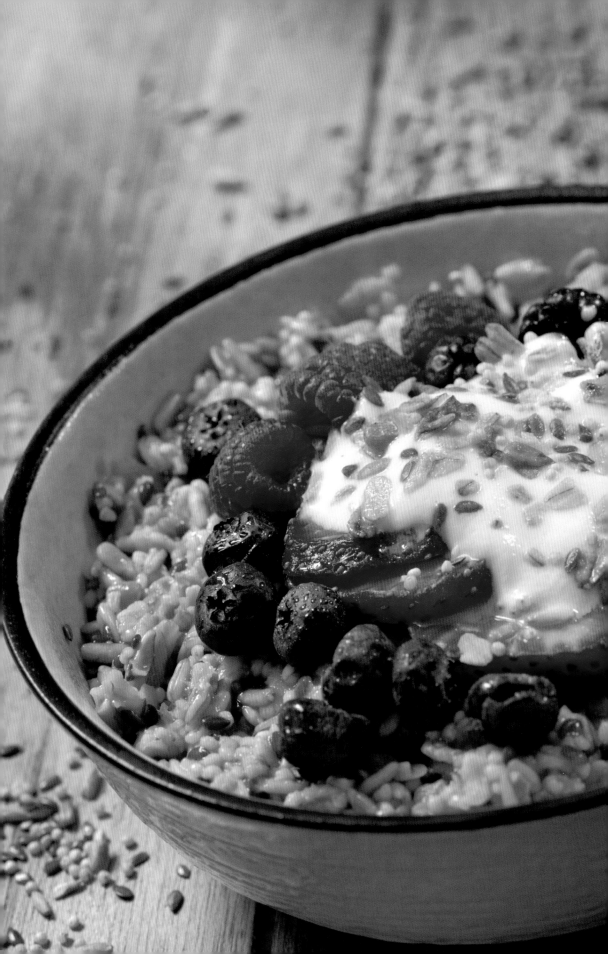

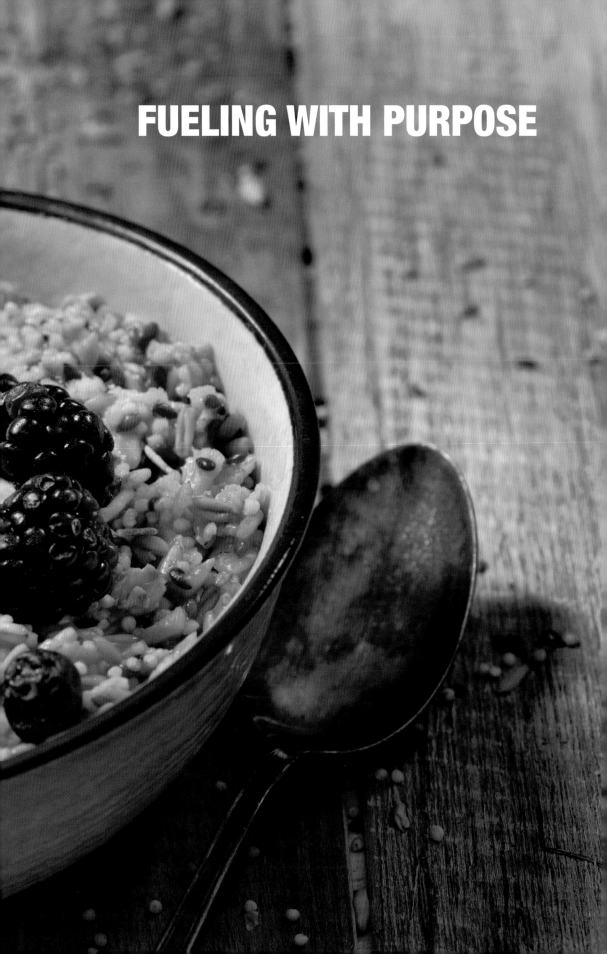

FUELING WITH PURPOSE

Recipes in *Finish Line Fueling* are to serve as a guide in empowering runners through simple fueling strategies in an effort to maximize the achievement of health, performance, and overall quality of life goals. View recipes as a learning opportunity that can be adapted based on individual goals and flavor preferences.

A simple grocery list of staple ingredients serves as the base of good fueling, yet each ingredient can be used in many different ways. This supports a busy, active lifestyle requiring the most efficient way to fuel the body. Each recipe focuses on the fundamental fueling concept—a balance between carbohydrates, protein, fat, and antioxidants—as often as possible. Through diet assessment using a tool such as Cronometer a runner can adjust the grocery list based on insufficient nutrient trends to better support maximizing everyday fueling needs.

Recipes are divided into foods commonly associated with meals, such as oatmeal for breakfast; however, there is no rule to what time of day a meal should be eaten. Delicious, savory oatmeal is a great source of fuel, be it breakfast, lunch, dinner, or a snack. Consider fueling with what the body communicates in need and strive for a balance of carbohydrates, protein, fat, antioxidants, and fluids at meals and snacks.

Tools and Appliances

Food Processor

My brand-name food processor is worth every penny of the initial hefty investment. It can be used for chopping vegetables, making a smooth puree, energy bars, dessert, soups, and more. A food processor has a motor that can handle the powerful grind needed for frozen bananas, tough to blend dates, and making a fine whole grain or nut-based flour.

Mini Power Blender

The easy cleanup and single serving use compared to a large-scale blender works great for an active, busy lifestyle.

Large-Rimmed Baking Sheets

Owning several baking sheets is well worth the investment. Save one baking sheet for hard to clean roasting, such as root vegetables and pumpkin seeds. Another baking sheet can be used for baking purposes.

32-Ounce Water Bottle

A water bottle labeled with 32-ounce measurements is perfect for shaking up a batch of sport drink.

Toaster

Storing bulk breads and pancakes keeps the day running smooth and efficient. A quick cycle in the toaster allows them to taste crisp and flavorful, like a fresh new batch.

Immersion or Stick Blender

A handheld blender is great for a quick soup puree, mashed potatoes, homemade pasta sauce, and pesto.

Cast-Iron Skillet

A well-seasoned cast-iron skillet is a great tool for even heat distribution and wonderful homemade breads.

Pizza Stone

The pizza stone works great for reheating leftovers, rejuvenating a nice texture or crunch. This tool can recreate a "fresh batch feel" to reheated homemade breads and pancakes. The pizza stone also works great for baking homemade pita bread.

Standing Mixer

The standing mixer is very much like the food processor and worth the investment. It offers a lot of hand-free moments in cooking that keeps meal prep efficient.

Large Stock Pot

A large study pot is great for bulk soup, stew, rice, quinoa, noodles, and more.

Parchment Paper

As much as a fast meal is needed, fast cleanup is even better. Cooking on parchment paper for dishes such fish, roasted vegetables, granola, and roasted pumpkin seeds offers a carefree cleanup for a time-crunched runner.

Crockpot

The crockpot is a convenient tool to handle every day cooking so you can be out running.

Grocery Purchasing Tips and Advice

Always keep fresh fruit within reach.

Fresh fruit is one of the simplest ways to provide the diet with quality carbohydrates and powerful antioxidants. The carbohydrate content of fruit supports stocking glycogen stores, which fuels endurance training. Antioxidants support a healthy immune system and the healing process required to prevent potential setbacks. Fresh fruit is also a fantastic substitute for poor quality sweet treats like candy and soda.

- Pair a banana with Greek yogurt for breakfast.
- Top a summer salad with fresh berries for lunch.
- Enjoy a ripe peach with dinner.
- Snack on a bowl of cherries for an evening treat.

Focus on vegetables as a building block.

While most vegetables lack the carbohydrate load of fresh fruit, they are a major building block of a high-quality diet. Vibrant colors like dark green leafy vegetables, a bright red bell pepper, and brilliant orange carrot offer an array of nutrients. Making effort to create colorful meals and snacks will support maximizing vitamins, minerals, and other beneficial nutrients to fuel great training and overall good health.

- Fresh celery supports electrolyte replacement after a high sweat loss run as a source of sodium, potassium, magnesium, calcium, and more.
- Bell peppers are great when eaten whole on the way to an afternoon meeting. Just toss the core as you would an apple.
- Snack on cherry tomatoes instead of chips during meal prep.
- Green leafy vegetables can act as the bed of most meals. Top them with the main meal ingredients including pasta, grilled chicken or salmon, eggs, chili, and quinoa with black beans and avocado.

Utilize the freezer.

The freezer is such a great opportunity to support a quick and easy, high quality meal. Stock the freezer with store bought or bulk-prepared plain brown rice and quinoa as well as discounted fruits and vegetables, just clean and chop before storing. It's easy to forget about leftovers in the refrigerator. Be sure to label and store leftovers in the freezer such as soups and stews, homemade breads, fresh farmer's market herbs, and even homemade cookies or cookie dough. The freezer can make mealtime fast, convenient, and budget friendly.

Skip the Packaged Meal Products

Explore the ingredients of desired prepackaged foods and investigate how to create the same product at home. This will save your budget and minimize undesirable ingredients that make the item shelf stable.

Protein Power

As the budget allows, aim to choose grass-fed meat and dairy as often as possible. Consider substituting half the amount of grass-fed meat in a recipe with beans to extend a pound of lean protein. Double up when purchasing sale priced wild caught fish. Simply store the extra fish in the freezer for future use. A few sale oysters shucked once every week or two are an extremely affordable way to boost B12, zinc, copper, iron, selenium, and iodine.

Toppings

Topping foods with a tablespoon of simple ingredients can truly boost the nutrition content significantly and fill nutrient gaps in everyday eating.

Nutritional Yeast
* B vitamins: B12, folate

Chia Seeds
* Omega-3, minerals, fiber

Pumpkin Seeds
* Minerals: iron, copper, zinc

Walnuts
* Omega-3, copper, manganese

Wheat Germ
* B vitamins, minerals, vitamin E

Almonds
* Vitamin E, biotin, copper

Flax Seed
* Omega-3, minerals, fiber, thiamin

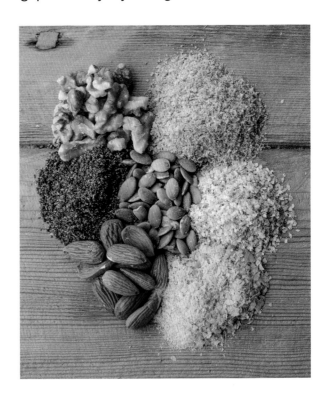

Base-Building Cooking Concepts

Before jumping into a hard effort, runners take measures to support a successful workout. Wearing the proper clothing and shoes, and having a good warm up, drills, and stretching allows a workout to go smooth and be most effective. Meal preparation should take similar form. With planning ahead, mealtime can be very efficient and effective, just like a successful tough workout.

Many recipes can be made in bulk to make future meal preparation smooth, easy, and energizing. Recipes such as homemade pitas, pancakes, and a simple batch of brown rice can be made in bulk to be divided out as immediate, tomorrow, and later. Immediate use will be served right away, tomorrow's portions can be stored in the refrigerator or pantry to be added to a meal in the next one to two days, and later use would be dated and stored in the freezer to be warmed and ready-to-eat.

Base Builders

Grains, Beans, and Pastas

Any time grains, beans, and pastas such as brown rice and quinoa are on the menu, prepare extra. For example, if a recipe calls for 2 cups of rice, prepare 4 cups of rice. This will allow the two additional cups of rice to make a quick meal the next day or freeze the two cups in a glass Tupperware dish or freezer bag to be reheated for future use.

Frozen Fruit and Vegetables

Frozen fruit is the perfect way to store fruit that may ripen before the opportunity to eat. Frozen fruit makes an excellent summer treat or smoothie addition. Purchasing discounted fruit or vegetables and freezing them for future use is a great way to fuel training and support the budget.

Meat

Skip cooked pre-packaged meats in the freezer section and simply prepare your own fresh meat for future use. While preparing a meal for immediate use, simply brown or grill an extra pound or two of meat. This can be added to a lunch meal the next day, or frozen for later use. This works well as a time crunch, easy protein source for future cooking

Fresh, Frozen, Canned

Choosing fresh or frozen ingredients is ideal. There are very few canned foods that should be part of mealtime. A few exceptions apply, one of which is in the purchase of beans. Beans are a great recipe boost as a source of protein, quality carbohydrates, filling fiber, and nutrient-rich energy source. Prepare them from scratch as often as possible. If fresh beans aren't an option, choose frozen beans as often as they are available. When choosing canned, look for those available in small boxes that are can size or choose BPA-free brands to limit BPA exposure.

Runner's Grocery Staples

Vegetables
Arugula
Asparagus
Beet
Broccoli
Bok Choy
Bell Peppers
Brussels Sprouts
Cabbage
Celery
Collard Greens
Vitamin D Mushrooms
Kale
Squash
Spinach
Sweet Potato
Tomato
White Potato
Zucchini

Fresh and Dried Fruit
Apple
Avocado
Banana
Cantaloupe
Date
Grape Juice
Kiwi
Oranges
Peach
Pineapple
Plum
Raisins
Strawberries

Beans and Lentils
Black Beans
Garbanzo Beans
Green Lentils
Kidney Beans
Lima Beans
Navy Beans
Soybeans

Meat
Chicken
Grass-fed Beef and Bison
Lamb
Lean Pork
Turkey

Seafood
Clams
Crab
Cod
Halibut
Lobster
Mussels
Sea Bass
Scallops
Salmon
Sardines
Shrimp
Tuna
Oysters

Dairy and Eggs
Omega-3 Eggs
Cow and Goat Milk
Grass-Fed Plain Yogurt
Plain Kefir
Raw Cheese
Cottage Cheese

Nuts and Seeds
Almonds
Brazil Nuts
Chia Seeds
Flax Seeds
Pumpkin Seeds
Quinoa
Tahini
Walnuts

Grains
Amaranth
Barley
Brown or Wild Rice
Buckwheat
Bulgur
Corn
Farro
Quinoa
Wheat Bran/Germ
Wheat, Spelt, Quinoa,
Buckwheat Noodles

Seasoning
Basil
Bay Leaf
Black Pepper
Cayenne Pepper
Salt
Chili Powder
Cinnamon
Cumin
Garlic
Ginger
Thyme
Turmeric
Sage
Pure Vanilla Extract

Miscellaneous
Blackstrap Molasses
Broth – chicken, vegetable,
seafood
Honey
Kimchi
Maca Root Powder
Maple Syrup
Nutritional Yeast
Sauerkraut

Flours
Bread
Brown Rice
Buckwheat
Oats
Rye
Self-Rising Spelt
Teff
White Whole Wheat

Recipe Key

All of the recipes in the pages ahead can be used as part of a high calorie or low calorie diet. Most often portions are suited to the lowest range of carbohydrates needs a runner should consume, with a general range of 50 to 70 grams. The runner with higher calorie needs should make effort to increase portions based on training demands and nutritional needs, or compliment the meal with options like fresh fruit, fruit juice, low fat milk, fresh bread, and kefir.

VEGETARIAN

Recipes labeled vegetarian do not contain meat in the form of beef, poultry, or lamb. They may contain fish, eggs, dairy, and honey.

VEGAN

Vegan recipes do not contain any ingredient sourced from animals.

GLUTEN-FREE

Gluten-free recipes are free of wheat, barley, and rye, but may contain gluten-free oats. Those who are sensitive to oats should avoid the recipe or replace gluten-free oats with a comparable alternative permitted in his or her diet. Be sure to compare labels to ensure a certified gluten-free label is available on any ingredient within a recipe for those highly sensitive or with a medical condition related to gluten.

PRE-RUN

Recipes labeled "pre-run" offer as a guide to pre-run meal options. Note that many recipes contain varied amounts of fiber. While fiber is a great part of a healthy diet, runners who feel sensitive to pre-run fiber will want to choose lower fiber pre-run options. If the diet is unaccustomed to fiber in general, slowly adding fiber to meals over time can often make them more tolerable.

ON-THE-RUN

"On-the-run" designates forms of fuel that can be used while running.

RECOVERY

Many of the recipes available would be suitable for recovery. To optimize recovery, aim for 10 to 30 grams of protein and roughly half of body weight in grams of carbohydrate. If a recipe does not meet recovery carbohydrate goals based on your specific weight, increase the serving or compliment the meal with other forms of carbohydrate such as fresh fruit, bread, or a walnut stuffed date. A recipe that is labeled recovery meets the low range of refueling needs for the average runner.

QUICK-TO-FIX

Meals that can be prepared in 30 minutes or less are considered quick-to-fix.

IRON, B12, MAGNESIUM, CALCIUM, VITAMIN D, PROBIOTICS

Any dish with 25 percent or more of iron, B12, calcium, and vitamin D will be labeled to support effort to maximize just a few key nutrients for runners. Probiotics are listed to support the thought process as to how a runner can get creative in adding them to the day in support of gut and immune system health.

Tip: Vitamin D synthesis occurs through sun exposure. However, effort in diet or through supplementation should be considered during low sun exposure months of the year.

HYDRATING

Recipes that support replacing fluids and electrolytes lost in sweat.

RECIPE SERVINGS AND NUTRITION FACTS

Servings are available as a guide to gain a general understanding of the nutrient content of a recipe. A single serving may meet the needs of one runner, while another may require two or more servings. The recipe servings and nutrition facts are beneficial as a reference to what ingredients carry nutrients and the combinations that can come together in meeting nutritional needs. Nutrition facts may vary related to the exact ingredients used, but serve as a practical guide.

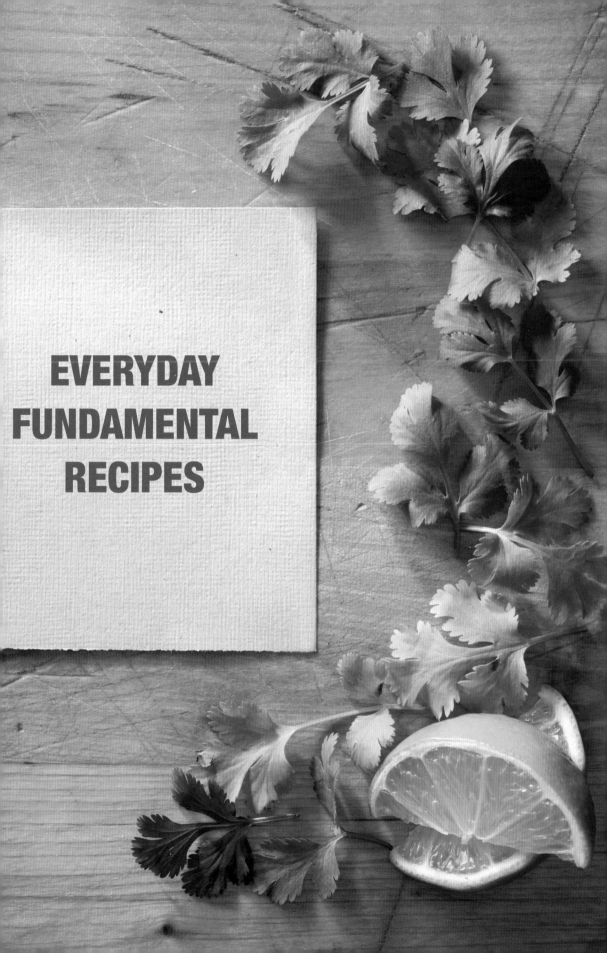

EVERYDAY
FUNDAMENTAL
RECIPES

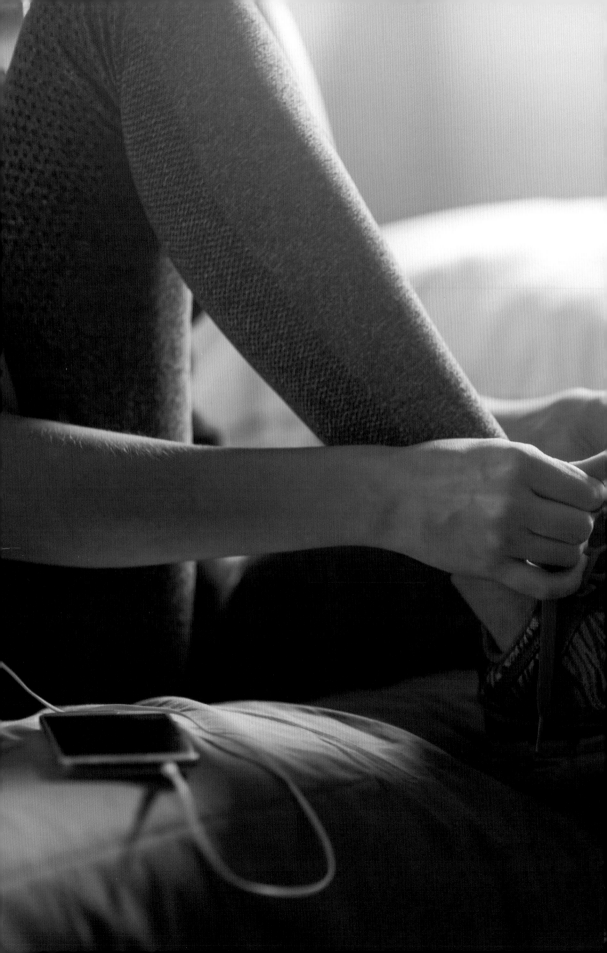

Breakfast

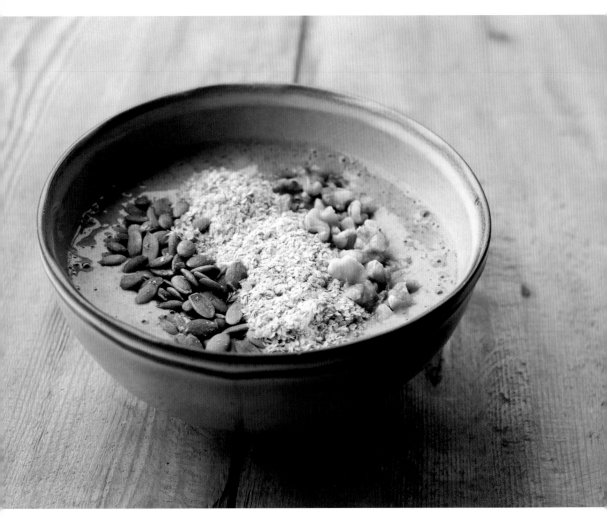

Smoothie Bowl

Finish Line Fueling

Smoothie Bowl

SERVES: 1
TOTAL TIME: 10 MINUTES

VEGAN, VEGETARIAN, QUICK-TO-FIX, MAGNESIUM, PRE-RUN, RECOVERY, HYDRATING

A smoothie bowl is a fantastic way to support hydration, recovery, and maximize micronutrients. Have fun with ingredients and toppings.

For a protein boost, consider adding a dollop or two of plain Greek or soy yogurt, a hard-boiled egg, or turkey bacon on the side. If this meal is used as a pre-race option, consider pairing it with a slice of toast with honey, fresh fruit, or yogurt for additional carbohydrates.

Ingredients:

1 c. coconut water
1 c. frozen banana chunks
1 c. fresh spinach
2 tbsp. wheat germ
2 tbsp. pumpkin seeds, (Sweet and Salty Pumpkin Seeds, page 203, works great for this recipe)
2 tbsp. walnuts
pinch of salt (optional)

Directions:

Blend coconut water, frozen banana, and spinach until smooth in a Magic Bullet or high power blender. Poor the smoothie mixture into a cereal bowl and top it with wheat germ, pumpkin seeds, and walnuts. Serve immediately and eat with a spoon.

Nutrition is approximately:

329 calories, 11 g fat, 1,413 mg potassium, 72 mg sodium, 59 g carbohydrate, 7 g fiber, 10 g protein, 59 percent vitamin A, 0 percent B12, 60 percent B6, 259 percent vitamin C, 0 percent vitamin D, 6 percent vitamin E, 11 percent calcium, 25 percent copper, 35 percent folate, 16 percent iron, 39 percent magnesium, 221 percent manganese, 12 percent niacin, 8 percent pantothenic acid, 25 percent phosphorus, 18 percent riboflavin, 22 percent selenium, 27 percent thiamin, 18 percent zinc

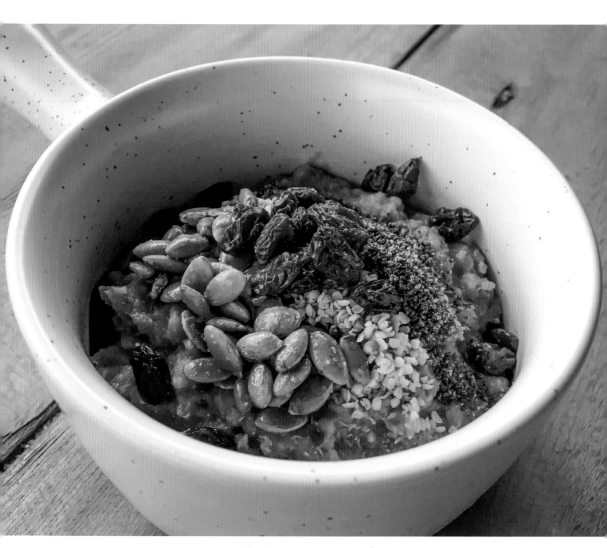

Quinoa Power Bowl

Quinoa Power Bowl

SERVES: 1
TOTAL TIME: 15 MINUTES

VEGETARIAN, VEGAN, QUICK-TO-FIX, RECOVERY, B12, IRON,
CALCIUM, MAGNESIUM, VITAMIN D, OMEGA-3

This power bowl is a fantastic source of fuel any time of day—breakfast, lunch, or dinner. The quinoa is prepared with fortified coconut milk as a vegan source of B12, calcium, and vitamin D.

To enjoy this meal as a pre-race option, reduce the amount of seeds by half and increase dried or fresh fruit. This will reduce the slow to digest fat content and increase the glycogen topping carbohydrate content. A high mileage runner should complement the warm porridge with options like fresh fruit, warm toast, or cup of milk within the 30 to 60 minutes after a demanding workout to better meet recovery needs.

Ingredients:

½ c. dry quinoa flakes
1¼ c. unsweetened, fortified coconut milk
½ tbsp. unsulfured blackstrap molasses
1 tbsp. ground flax seeds
1 tbsp. hemp seeds
1 tbsp. pumpkin seeds
2 to 3 dashes cinnamon
1 to 2 pinches salt
maple syrup, honey, or agave syrup (optional)

Directions:

In a small saucepan bring coconut milk to a slow boil. Add the quinoa stirring constantly for about 30 seconds and turn off heat. Add the molasses, cinnamon, and salt. Top with hemp, pumpkin, and flax seed and serve.

Nutrition is approximately:

439 calories, 18 g fat, 528 mg potassium, 0 mg cholesterol, 296 mg sodium, 57 g carb, 9 g fiber, 14 g protein, 13 percent vitamin A, 63 percent B12, 12 percent B6, 3 percent vitamin C, 38 percent vitamin D, 3 percent vitamin E, 27 percent calcium, 15 percent copper, 10 percent folate, 36 percent iron, 37 percent magnesium, 38 percent manganese, 2 percent niacin, 1 percent pantothenic acid, 44 percent phosphorus, 85 percent riboflavin, 15 percent selenium, 12 percent thiamin, 15 percent zinc, 1.15 g omega-3

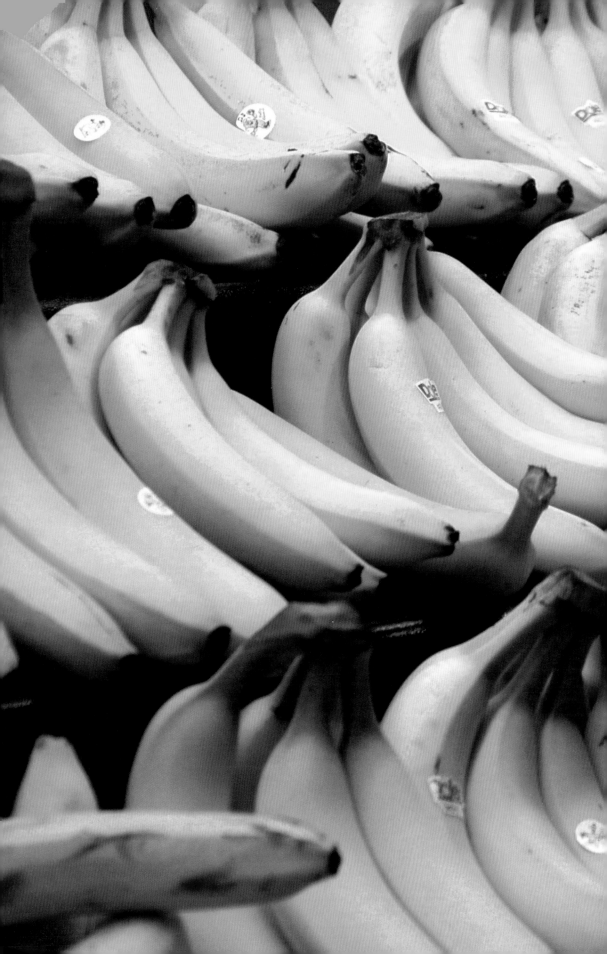

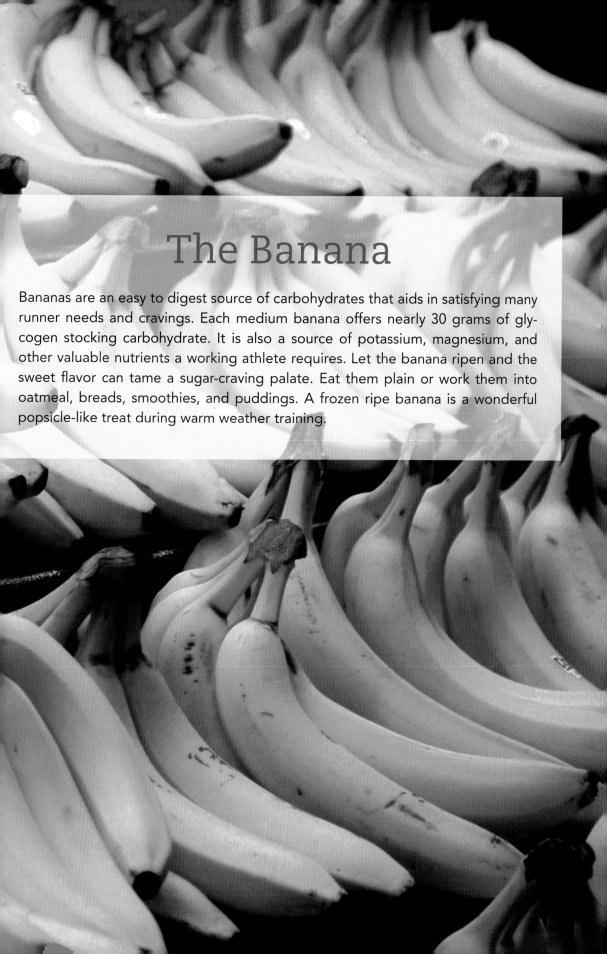

The Banana

Bananas are an easy to digest source of carbohydrates that aids in satisfying many runner needs and cravings. Each medium banana offers nearly 30 grams of glycogen stocking carbohydrate. It is also a source of potassium, magnesium, and other valuable nutrients a working athlete requires. Let the banana ripen and the sweet flavor can tame a sugar-craving palate. Eat them plain or work them into oatmeal, breads, smoothies, and puddings. A frozen ripe banana is a wonderful popsicle-like treat during warm weather training.

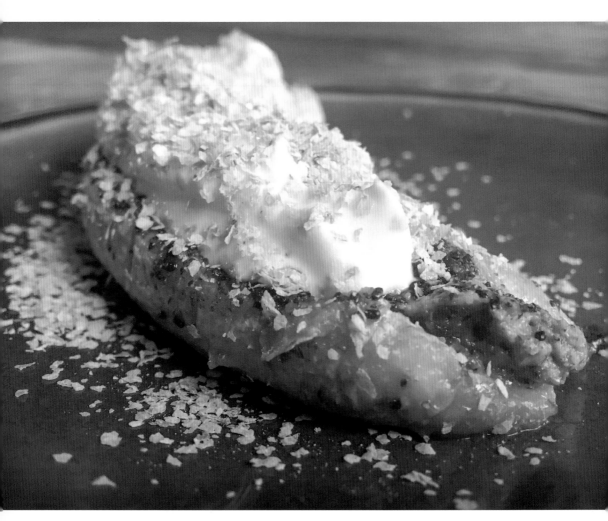

Baked Banana

Baked Banana

SERVES 1
TOTAL TIME: 25 MINUTES

VEGETARIAN, VEGAN, QUICK-TO-FIX, PRE-RUN,
POST-RUN, MAGNESIUM, PROBIOTICS, OMEGA-3

Baked bananas can make a satisfying breakfast, pre-race fuel, recovery option, or evening snack. A heavy training runner may need to pair this baked banana recipe with additional carbohydrate sources if used for pre-race or recovery fueling, aiming closer to roughly half of body weight in grams of carbohydrate as tolerated. Great options include adding additional honey, yogurt, to wheat germ or pair it with a glass of milk, kefir, juice, or toast.

Ingredients:

1 large banana
1 tbsp. almond butter
½ tsp. ground chia seeds
1 tsp. honey
¼ c. plain grass-fed whole milk
    Greek yogurt
1 tsp. wheat germ

Directions:

Preheat oven to 375 degrees. Place the banana on a baking sheet topped with parchment paper. Slice halfway through the banana. Fill the banana slice with the almond butter. Top the almond butter with chia seeds. Coat the outer flesh of the banana with honey, smoothing the honey out with your finger such that any exposed banana will be coated in honey. Bake the banana for 15 to 20 minutes. Cool slightly and top with plain Greek yogurt and wheat germ.

Nutrition is approximately:

319 calories, 12 g fat, 26 mg sodium, 612 mg potassium, 46 g carbohydrate, 9 g fiber, 13 g protein, 2 percent vitamin A, 10 percent B12, 40 percent B6, 20 percent vitamin C, 0 percent vitamin D, 18 percent vitamin E, 17 percent calcium, 16 percent copper, 13 percent folate, 12 percent iron, 25 percent magnesium, 76 percent manganese, 8 percent niacin, 5 percent pantothenic acid, 17 percent phosphorus, 15 percent riboflavin, 10 percent selenium, 14 percent thiamin, 11 percent zinc, 273 mg omega-3

Savory Maca Oats

SERVES: 1
TOTAL TIME: 20 MINUTES

PRE-RUN, RECOVERY, GLUTEN-FREE, LOW-CALORIE,
IRON, OMEGA-3, QUICK-TO-FIX

Savory maca oats is a comfort food recipe that will quickly become a craved favorite. Maca root powder offers a pleasant nutty flavor to the oats. The root is often associated with its adaptogenic properties to aid the body in managing stress and cortisol. It is rich in iron, iodine, potassium, and calcium.

To optimize this dish for pre-run, post-run, or high calorie needs complement the dish with fresh fruit, low-fat milk, or an extra helping of oats to meet individual carbohydrate goals.

Ingredients:

1 c. spinach
¼ tsp. horseradish
1 large omega-3 egg
1 large egg white
1 slice turkey bacon, diced
6 cherry tomatoes, halved
½ c. gluten-free quick oats
¾ c. boiling water
⅛ tsp. salt
1 tsp. maca powder
½ tsp. butter, as needed for frying
    egg (optional)

Directions:

Combine the boiling water and oats in a small bowl and cover. Let the oats rest until soft and the water is well absorbed. Add maca powder and salt.

Whisk together the egg white and horseradish in a small bowl and set aside. In a skillet over medium heat, toss together the turkey bacon, spinach, and tomatoes until the tomatoes just begin to soften, spinach begins to wilt, and bacon is fully cooked. Place the cooked vegetable mixture on top of the maca oats.

Cook the scrambled eggs in the warm skillet. Place the cooked egg white on top of the vegetable mixture. Lastly, cook the whole egg for about 2½ minutes on each side, leaving a soft yolk for an over easy egg. Top the oatmeal with the egg and serve immediately.

Tip: Those who are on hormone-altering medications, who are pregnant, or who have high blood pressure should consult their doctor before using maca root powder.

Nutrition per recipe is approximately:

390 calories, 16 g fat, 962 mg potassium, 45 g carbohydrate, 11 g fiber, 20 g protein, 122 percent vitamin A, 8 percent B12, 63 percent B6, 89 percent vitamin C, 0 percent vitamin D, 30 percent vitamin E, 29 percent calcium, 60 percent folate, 61 percent iron, 31 percent magnesium, 88 percent manganese, 48 percent niacin, 12 percent pantothenic acid, 44 percent riboflavin, 28 percent selenium, 52 percent thiamin, 15 percent zinc, 306 mg omega

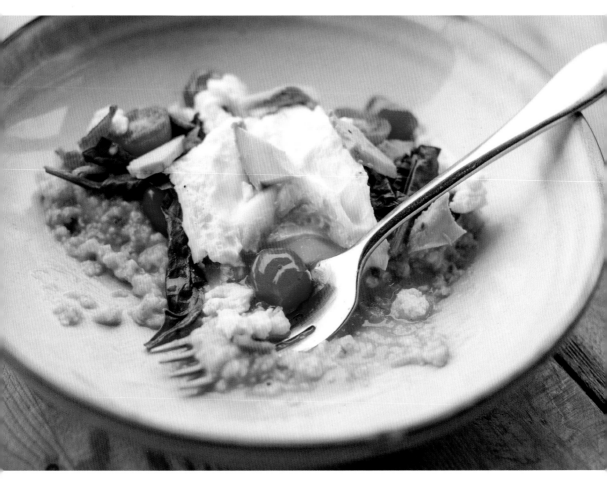

Savory Maca Oats

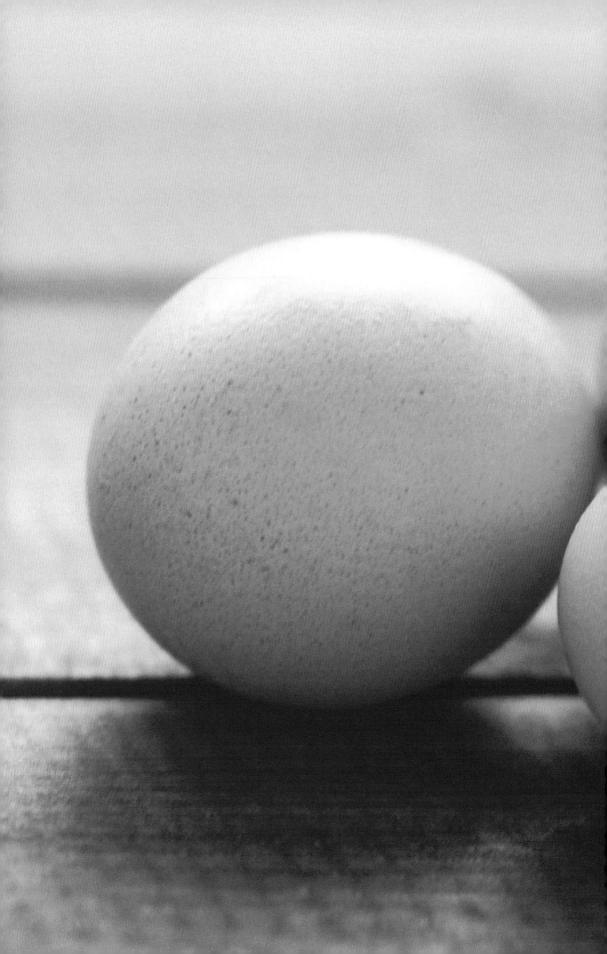

The Egg

Eggs are a fantastic fuel for a training runner. They are versatile, easy to make, and chock full of nutrients. Standout nutrients include B12, iodine, selenium, choline, and omega-3. Iodine-rich foods support the thyroid health of a heavy training runner.

Be creative with the egg. Swap the typical sugar-rich oatmeal topping for a savory and satisfying soft egg yolk. Scramble eggs with horseradish as a potato topping. Combine eggs with turmeric and veggies for an anti-inflammatory boost. My personal favorite egg meal is an egg or two on top of a warm garlic butter spinach salad. Hardboiled egg, tomato, and avocado topped on toast or a rice cake with salt and nutritional yeast works great for snacking.

Just remember that many of the beneficial nutrients lie in the yolk of the egg. Purchase omega-3 eggs for a source of omega-3 fatty acids.

Iron Spice Pancakes

SERVES 4
TOTAL TIME: 30 MINUTES

VEGETARIAN, PRE-RUN, POST-RUN, IRON, OMEGA-3

Pancakes just got kicked up a notch for the runner looking to boost iron intake while fueling performance. Ginger supports soothing pre-race stomach jitters or a post-run poor appetite. Cinnamon honey butter can be a means to support topping off the glycogen stores of a nervous, poor pre-race appetite. Pair this meal with a fresh orange or orange juice as a source of vitamin C to support iron absorption and a hard-boiled egg for a boost or protein. Save any leftovers for future toasting.

Ingredients:

1 c. spelt flour
⅔ c. teff flour
¾ c. pumpkin (or butternut squash) puree
1 tsp. baking soda
¼ tsp. salt
½ tsp. fresh grated ginger
¼ tsp. cinnamon
1 large omega-3 egg
1 c. milk
¼ c. orange juice
1 tbsp. unsalted butter

Cinnamon Honey Butter (Optional Topping)

1 tbsp. butter, softened
¼ tsp. cinnamon
¼ c. honey

Tip: Let the pancake slowly cook over lower heat and avoid making large pancakes. This will offer a nice fluffy rise to the pancake.

Directions:

Preheat skillet or griddle to medium-low heat. Combine all dry ingredients in a medium bowl. Add the pumpkin puree, egg, ginger, milk, and juice. Stir to combine. Lightly spread some of the butter over the warm skillet or griddle to lightly coat; reserve the rest of pad of butter. Gently spread a spoonful of pancake batter on the buttered hot skillet. When ¼ to ½ inch in from pancake edge starts to look formed, flip the pancake. Remove from skillet or griddle when the other side of pancake has nicely browned. Run the pad of butter over the skillet again to gently coat between each pancake as needed.

Mash and stir the cinnamon honey butter ingredients together in a small bowl. Top each pancake with cinnamon honey butter.

Makes approximately eight 6-inch pancakes.

Nutrition per two pancakes is approximately:

298 calories, 6.4 g of fat, 187 mg sodium, 264 mg potassium, 48 g of carb, 8.2 g fiber, 11 g protein, 148 percent vitamin A, 7 percent B12, 4.3 percent B-6, 12 percent vitamin C, 10.4 percent vitamin D, 0.6 percent vitamin E, 17 percent calcium, 5.7 percent copper, 3 percent folate, 26.6 percent iron, 4.8 percent magnesium, 6.8 percent manganese, 0.8

percent niacin, 3 percent pantothenic acid, 8.8 percent phosphorus, 9.6 percent riboflavin, 4.2 percent selenium, 2.1 percent thiamin, 3.1 percent zinc

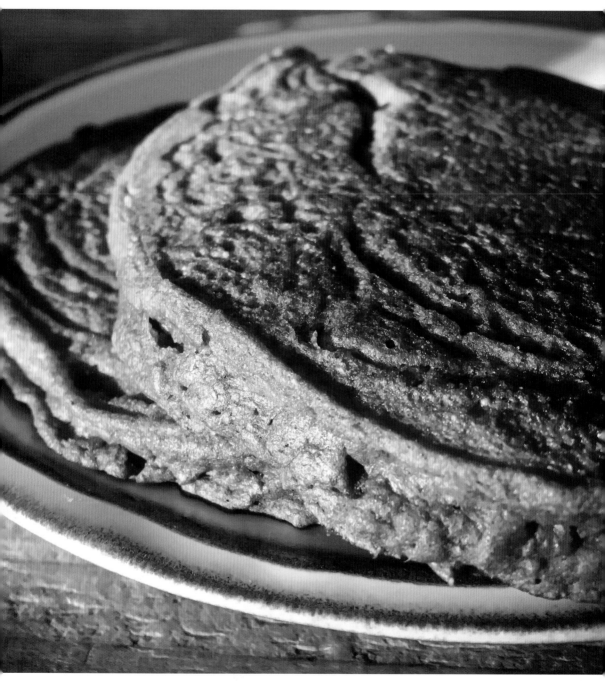

Iron Spice Pancake

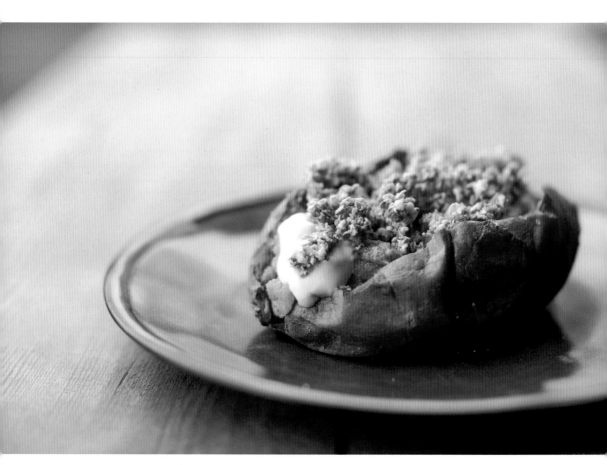

Almond Granola Sweet Potato

Almond Granola Sweet Potato

SERVES 1
TOTAL TIME: 5 MINUTES

GLUTEN-FREE, VEGETARIAN, VEGAN, QUICK-TO-FIX, PROBIOTICS

Take any opportunity to bake extra sweet potatoes. If a dinner meal calls for four baked potatoes, make six. This will make a breakfast potato stuffed with almond butter, Greek yogurt, granola, and maybe even a drizzle of honey or maple syrup a carefree change from the typical breakfast from a box. Don't forget to enjoy the nutrient dense potato skin!

Ingredients:

1 large sweet potato, baked
1 tbsp. almond butter
a few dashes of cinnamon, nutmeg, or allspice (optional)
¼ c. plain grass-fed whole milk yogurt
¼ c. buckwheat oat granola (see page 175)
salt to taste

Directions:

Warm a leftover sweet potato in the microwave. If baking fresh, pre-heat the oven to 425 degrees. Wash a sweet potato and poke it with a fork on several sides. Place the potato on a baking sheet and bake the potato for about 45–60 minutes until it reaches the desired softness. I recommend a potato that is extra soft and sweet.

Slice the potato down the center. Fill the potato with the almond butter, and any spice desired. Top with yogurt and granola. Serve immediately.

Nutrition is approximately:

437 calories, 15 g fat, 64 g carbohydrate, 222 mg sodium, 1115 mg potassium, 10 fiber, 15 g protein, 216 percent vitamin A, 10 percent B12, 37 percent B6, 43 percent vitamin C, 1 percent vitamin D, 30 percent vitamin E, 20 percent calcium, 47 percent copper, 8 percent folate, 20 percent iron, 35 percent magnesium, 93 percent manganese, 24 percent niacin, 41 percent pantothenic acid, 31 percent phosphorus, 22 percent riboflavin, 8 percent selenium, 24 percent thiamin, 22 percent zinc

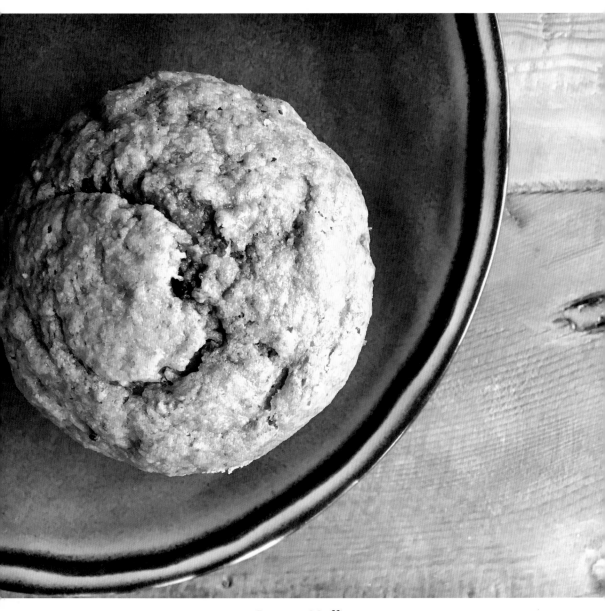

Banana Muffin

Banana Muffins

SERVES 9
TOTAL TIME: 35 MINUTES

VEGETARIAN, GLUTEN-FREE, OMEGA-3

Banana muffins are an easy go-to that can serve many roles. Something as simple as a pre-race muffin with fruit, yogurt, honey, and sports drink about 1 to 2 hours before a race start will support fueling a strong finish. Snack on a single muffin with yogurt 45 to 60 minutes before late day workout. Pair a muffin with kefir and fresh fruit within 30 minutes of a tough workout.

Ingredients:

6 tbsp. soft butter, unsalted
½ c. honey
2 large omega-3 eggs
2 c. gluten-free oat flour
½ tsp. salt
1 tsp. baking soda
1 c. mashed over-ripe bananas or
    about 3 medium bananas, mashed
2 tbsp. ground chia seeds
3 tbsp. plain kefir

Directions:

Preheat oven to 350 degrees. Combine oat flour, salt, chia seed, and baking soda and set aside. Mix butter and honey until well combined. Add eggs and mix to combine. Add oat flour mixture to combine. Fold mashed banana and kefir into mixture. Evenly distribute between 9 muffin cups or a lightly butter coated muffin pan. Bake for about 25 minutes. Makes 9 large muffins.

Tip: Remove the muffins looking slightly under cooked vs. overcooking them for a nice moist center.

Nutrition per muffin is approximately:

281 calories, 11 g fat, 166 mg potassium, 281 mg sodium, 39 g carbohydrate, 3 g fiber, 6 g protein, 8 percent vitamin A, 2 percent B12, 13 percent B6, 7 percent vitamin C, 2 percent vitamin D, 2 percent vitamin E, 4 percent calcium, 7 percent copper, 5 percent folate, 8 percent iron, 13 percent magnesium, 56 percent manganese, 3 percent niacin, 1 percent pantothenic acid, 15 percent phosphorus, 6 percent riboflavin, 14 percent selenium, 13 percent thiamin, 7 percent zinc, 344 mg omega-3

Turmeric Egg Scramble

SERVES 1
TOTAL TIME: 15 MINUTES

VEGETARIAN, GLUTEN-FREE, B12, VITAMIN D, OMEGA-3

Slip turmeric into a morning egg scramble to take advantage of the anti-inflammatory properties it carries. Serving turmeric eggs with an assortment of brilliant colorful vegetables boosts the antioxidant and micronutrient potential. Pair this otherwise low carbohydrate dish with potato, toast, brown rice, fresh fruit, or yogurt to supply necessary glycogen stocking carbohydrates.

Ingredients:

2 large egg whites
2 tbsp. low fat milk
¼ tsp. turmeric
1 loose cup of green leafy vegetable
  (arugula, spinach, or kale)
¼ c. cherry tomatoes, halved
⅔ c. vitamin D mushrooms, chopped
1 tsp. olive oil
salt and pepper to taste

Directions:

Whisk together the egg whites, milk, turmeric, and pinch of salt in a small bowl and set aside. Combine olive oil, and vegetables in a medium skillet over medium heat and sauté for 3 to 5 minutes.

When the tomato and mushrooms start to turn soft add the egg mixture. Using a spatula, toss the vegetable and egg mixture until the egg is fully cooked and serve.

Tip: Turmeric eggs are delicious paired with horseradish cream.

Tip: Turmeric in food is considered safe and can be added to basic cooking often. Medicinal doses of turmeric can interfere with some blood thinners, stomach acid reducers, and diabetes medications.

Nutrition per recipe is approximately:

200 calories, 10 g fat, 349 mg potassium, 201 mg sodium, 11 g carbohydrate, 2 g fiber, 17 g protein, 25 percent vitamin A, 14 percent B12, 9 percent B6, 47 percent vitamin C, 123 percent vitamin D, 4 percent vitamin E, 10 percent calcium, 9 percent copper, 14 percent folate, 11 percent iron, 5 percent magnesium, 7 percent manganese, 10 percent niacin, 9 percent pantothenic acid, 18 percent phosphorus, 26 percent riboflavin, 8 percent selenium, 4 percent thiamin, 8 percent zinc, 225 mg omega-3

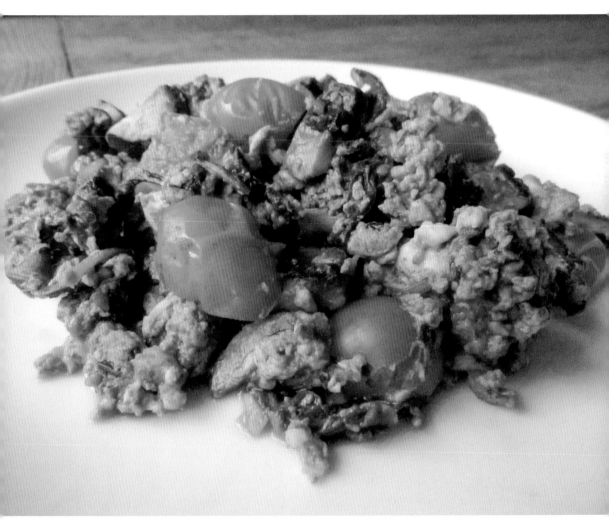

Turmeric Egg Scramble

Sauces and Breads

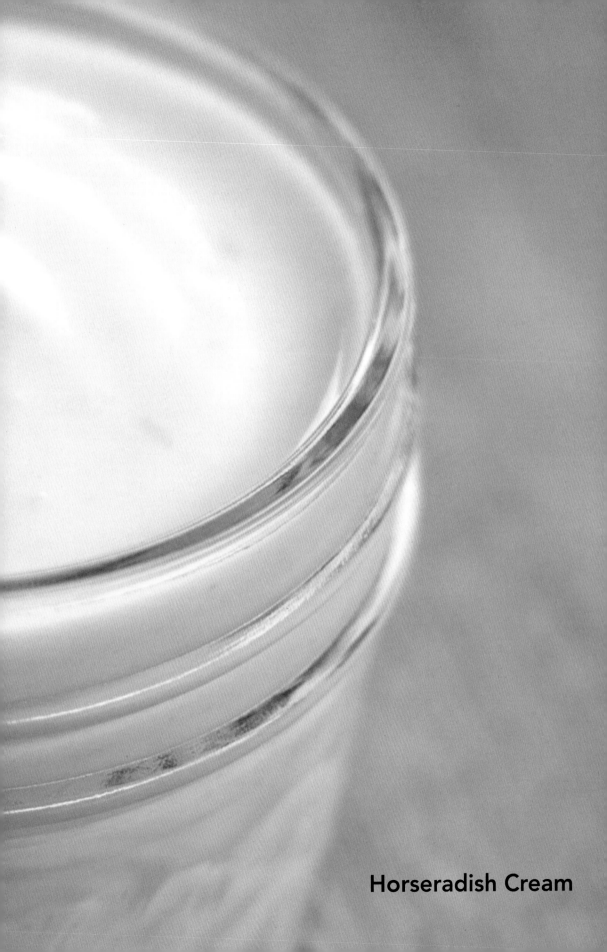

Horseradish Cream

Sauces

Many of the sauces and dressings that fill the grocery aisles are full of added ingredients the diet can do without. Create recipe enhancing sauces and toppings with fresh ingredients that will fuel health and training.

Horseradish Cream

SERVES 4
TOTAL TIME: 5 MINUTES

VEGETARIAN, GLUTEN-FREE, QUICK-TO-FIX, PROBIOTICS

Horseradish is a great way to add a little kick to mealtime. On top of eggs, sauerkraut, and meats are just a few favorite ways to incorporate horseradish in the day. The potent antioxidant-rich ingredient contains anti-microbial, anti-bacterial, anti-inflammatory properties to support fighting harmful bacteria and inflammation. Keep a small Tupperware of horseradish cream in the refrigerator for an easy mealtime flavor enhancing addition.

Ingredients:

¼ c. low fat grass-fed sour cream (or whole milk yogurt)
1 tsp. horseradish
1 tsp. lemon juice
salt and pepper to taste

Directions:

Combine all ingredients in a small bowl and serve.

Tip: Great with fish, beef, vegetables, and as a sandwich topping. The options with this sauce are limitless. Add a touch of ketchup for a Thousand Island dressing flavor.

Nutrition per serving is approximately:

22 calories, 2 g fat, 28 mg potassium, 1 g carbohydrate, 0 g fiber, 0.5 g protein, 1 percent vitamin A, 1 percent B12, 0 percent B6, 4 percent vitamin C, 0 percent vitamin D, 0 percent vitamin E, 2 percent calcium, 0 percent copper, 1 percent folate, 0 percent iron, 1 percent magnesium, 0 percent manganese, 1 percent niacin, 1 percent pantothenic acid, 2 percent phosphorus, 2 percent riboflavin, 1 percent selenium, 1 percent thiamin, 1 percent zinc

Avocado Cream

SERVES 5
TOTAL TIME: 5 MINUTES

VEGETARIAN, GLUTEN-FREE, QUICK-TO-FIX

Avocado cream is a nourishing topping for sandwiches, tacos, a rice bowl, salad, or on warm toast with fresh tomato and nutritional yeast. It supplies beneficial oleic fatty acids compared to a typical mayonnaise or stand-alone sour cream. For a thinner consistency, add a touch of water, extra juice, or yogurt and pinch of salt.

Ingredients:

1 ripe avocado
2 tbsp. low fat sour cream or
    plain yogurt
½ lime, juiced
pinch of salt

Directions:

Blend all ingredients together in a small food processor until smooth.

Nutrition per serving is approximately:

68 calories, 5.5 g fat, 184 mg potassium, 5 mg sodium, 4 g carbohydrate, 3 g fiber, 2 g protein, 2 percent vitamin A, 0 percent B12, 2 percent B6, 17 percent vitamin C, 0 percent vitamin D, 0 percent vitamin E, 1 percent calcium, 8 percent copper, 4 percent folate, 1 percent iron, 3 percent magnesium, 2 percent manganese, 2 percent niacin, 5 percent pantothenic acid, 2 percent phosphorus, 2 percent riboflavin, 0 percent selenium, 1 percent thiamin, 1 percent zinc

Avocado Pesto

SERVES 5
TOTAL TIME: 5 MINUTES

VEGETARIAN, VEGAN, GLUTEN-FREE, QUICK-TO-FIX

Toss a batch of avocado pesto with pasta and fresh cut vegetables for a very fast carbohydrate-rich meal that can work great as a lunch salad, quick dinner, or pre-race meal. Substitute basil with cilantro and lime for lemon for a pleasant southwest flavor.

Ingredients:

1 avocado
1 tbsp. olive oil
⅓ c. fresh basil
2 tbsp. lemon juice
½ c. water
½ tsp. salt

Directions:

Blend all ingredients in a food processor or blender until smooth.

Nutrition per serving is approximately:

125 calories, 11 g fat, 298 mg potassium, 267 mg sodium, 7 g carbohydrate, 4 g fiber, 2 g protein, 6 percent vitamin A, 0 percent B12, 4 percent B6, 32 percent vitamin C, 0 percent vitamin D, 2 percent vitamin E, 1 percent calcium, 13 percent copper, 8 percent folate, 1 percent iron, 5 percent magnesium, 6 percent manganese, 3 percent niacin, 7 percent pantothenic acid, 3 percent phosphorus, 3 percent riboflavin, 0 percent selenium, 1 percent thiamin, 2 percent zinc

Cinnamon Honey Butter

SERVES 5
TOTAL TIME: 5 MINUTES

VEGETARIAN, GLUTEN-FREE, QUICK-TO-FIX, PRE-RUN, RECOVERY

Cinnamon honey butter is a nice way to slip a sweet topping and treat into mealtime without surrendering to the bowl of candy or sleeve of cookies. The honey topping also serves as a source of easy to consume carbohydrates for when appetite is down or calorie demands are difficult to achieve. Add a coat of honey butter to pre-race or recovery eating to support meeting carbohydrate goals when needed.

Ingredients:

¼ c. honey
1 tbsp. butter
⅛ tsp. cinnamon

Directions:

Stir together all ingredients and serve, or place in an airtight container and store in the refrigerator for future use.

Nutrition per serving is approximately:

90 calories, 3 g fat, 12 mg potassium, 1 mg sodium, 18 g carbohydrate, 0 g fiber, 0 g protein, 2 percent vitamin A, 0 percent B12, 0 percent B6, 0 percent vitamin C, 0 percent vitamin D, 0 percent vitamin E, 0 percent calcium, 1 percent copper, 0 percent folate, 1 percent iron, 0 percent magnesium, 2 percent manganese, 0 percent niacin, 0 percent pantothenic acid, 0 percent phosphorus, 1 percent riboflavin, 0 percent selenium, 0 percent thiamin, 0 percent zinc

Mustard Cream

SERVES 1
TOTAL TIME: 5 MINUTES

VEGETARIAN, GLUTEN-FREE, QUICK-TO-FIX, PROBITOTICS

Homemade or commercial mustard serves as a source of turmeric and electrolyte replacing sodium. Adding yogurt offers as a source of probiotics as well as a creamy flavor that works great as a mayonnaise-like sandwich topping. Make this for a single serving sandwich or prepare a bulk batch and store it for later use.

Ingredients:

2 tsp. yellow mustard
2 tbsp. plain yogurt

Directions:

Stir together all ingredients and serve, or place in an airtight container and store in the refrigerator for future use.

Nutrition per serving is approximately:

42 calories, 1 g fat, 147 mg potassium, 152 mg sodium, 5 g carbohydrate, 0 g fiber, 3 g protein, 1 percent vitamin A, 5 percent B12, 2 percent B6, 1 percent vitamin C, 0 percent vitamin D, 1 percent vitamin E, 11 percent calcium, 1 percent copper, 2 percent folate, 1 percent iron, 3 percent magnesium, 2 percent manganese, 1 percent niacin, 4 percent pantothenic acid, 9 percent phosphorus, 7 percent riboflavin, 8 percent selenium, 2 percent thiamin, 4 percent zinc

Everyday Dressing

SERVES 4
TOTAL TIME: 5 MINUTES

VEGETARIAN, VEGAN, GLUTEN-FREE, QUICK-TO-FIX

Many claim unfiltered apple cider vinegar can help clear lactic acid, reduce muscle sore-ness, and support recovery. While more research is needed to support the role of apple cider vinegar related to performance, the powerful vinegar has many health benefits. Apple cider vinegar supports insulin sensitivity and healthy blood sugar. The pleasantly powerful flavor allows for healthy portion control offering wonderful flavor in every bite for a no calorie cost.

Olive and avocado oils offer a source of healthy fatty acids and inflammation fighting polyphenols. Garlic and lemon juice also carry antioxidant properties to support a healthy immune system. Keep a jar of this powerful dressing on hand to add healthful flavor to mealtime.

Ingredients:

¼ c. unfiltered apple cider vinegar
2 tbsp. lemon juice
2 tbsp. olive or avocado oil
⅛ tsp. salt and pepper to taste
1 clove garlic, minced
2 tbsp. water

Directions:

Combine all ingredients in a Mason jar or small container. Place lid on the jar and shake vigorously. Serve right away or place in the refrigerator to let the flavor develop.

Nutrition per serving is approximately:

62 calories, 7 g fat, 23 mg potassium, 63 mg sodium, 1 g carbohydrate, 0 g fiber, 0 g protein, 0 percent vitamin A, 0 percent B12, 1 percent B6, 6 percent vitamin C, 0 percent vitamin D, 4 percent vitamin E, 1 percent calcium, 0 percent copper, 0 percent folate, 0 percent iron, 1 percent magnesium, 3 percent manganese, 0 percent niacin, 0 percent pantothenic acid, 1 percent phosphorus, 3 percent riboflavin, 0 percent selenium, 0 percent thiamin, 0 percent zinc

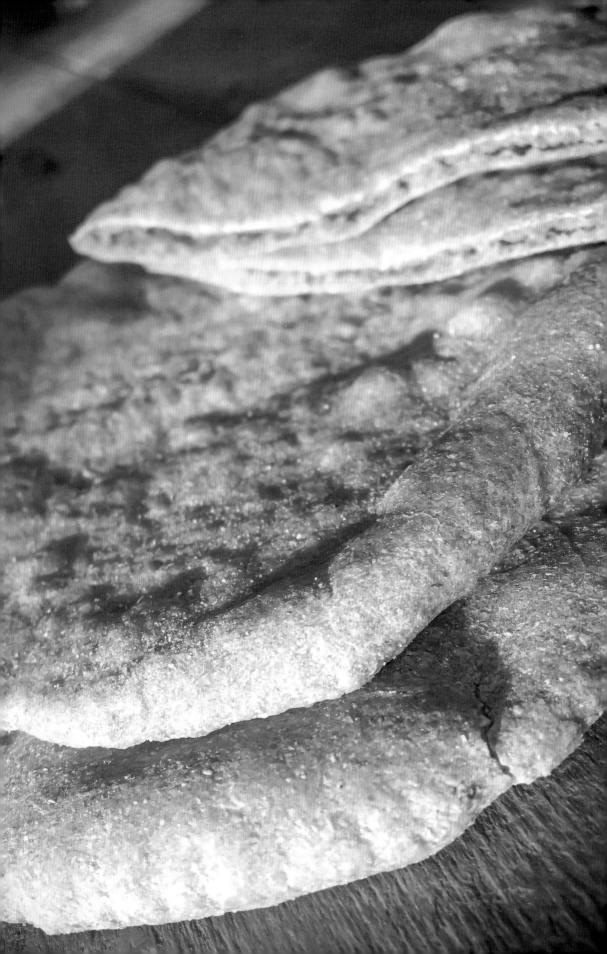

Bread

Many runners cut bread from the diet because they associate unwanted symptoms to the carbohydrate source. While it is true some runners suffer from gluten sensitivity, intolerance, or an allergy, the culprit in bread may not be the actual gluten. Majority of the breads in the aisles of the grocery store contain many ingredients, including forms of corn, soy, and preservatives. The cause of the undesirable symptoms may be related to ingredients not related to gluten.

Making breads at home from scratch allows for greater control of easy to digest ingredients and eliminates the undesirable additions that keep bread shelf-stable. Store pancakes, pitas, and breads in the freezer to be used as needed if they mold faster than they are eaten.

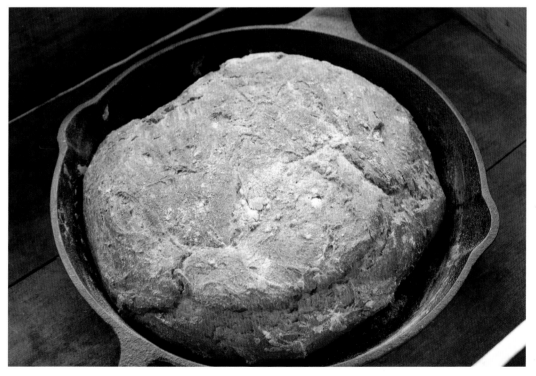

Everyday Grain Chia Bread

Spelt Pita Bread

SERVES 12
TOTAL TIME: 2.5 HOURS

VEGETARIAN, VEGAN, PRE-RUN, RECOVERY

Pita bread is great for sandwich stuffing, making mini pizzas, serving beside a fresh salad, or topping with butter and honey. Spelt contains gluten, but is often better tolerate and easier to digest compared to wheat counterparts. The higher protein content, digestibility, and source of vitamins, minerals, and fiber make spelt a great everyday flour of choice.

Ingredients:

1 packet fast-acting yeast
1½ c. warm water
3½ c. spelt flour
1 tsp. olive oil

Directions:

Dissolve the yeast in warm water and let sit for about 5 minutes. The yeast water should begin to foam as a sign the yeast is activated. If the water is too hot the yeast will die. Combine the flour and yeast activated water. Knead the dough for about 8 to 10 minutes. Add the olive oil to a medium bowl, creating an olive oil coating on the bowl. Place the dough in the bowl. Flip the dough over such that each side of the dough has a little coating of oil from the bowl. Cover the dough with a clean towel and place it in a warm location. I often preheat the oven to 150 degrees, turn off the oven, place the dough on a cookie sheet in the slightly warmed oven to support a warm location, and let dough rise.

The dough should double in size in about 1 to 2 hours.

Preheat the oven to 500 degrees. Place a pizza or baking stone in lower third of the oven. Divide the dough into 10 equal pieces and flatten slightly with your hands. Place the dough on a baking sheet and cover with a clean cloth. Let it sit for about 10 minutes.

Lightly flour a clean surface and roll the individual dough on the floured surface into about a 6-inch circle.

Place two round pita dough on the hot stone and bake for about 3 to 5 minutes, until the bread starts to balloon. Flip the pita and bake another couple minutes. Don't worry if the pita does not always balloon. Serve immediately or cool and store in an airtight container.

Nutrition per serving is approximately:

145 calories, 1 g fat, 325 mg sodium, 160 mg K, 31 g carbohydrate, 4 g fiber, 6 g protein, 0 percent vitamin A, 0 percent B12, 5 percent B6, 0 percent vitamin C, 0 percent vitamin D, 2 percent vitamin E, 1 percent calcium, 12 percent copper, 4 percent folate, 11 percent iron, 15 percent magnesium, 62 percent manganese, 15 percent niacin, 2 percent pantothenic acid, 17 percent phosphorus, 2 percent riboflavin, 7 percent selenium, 8 percent thiamin, 10 percent zinc

Everyday Grain Chia Bread

SERVES 24
TOTAL TIME: 10 HOURS

VEGETARIAN, VEGAN, PRE-RUN, RECOVERY, OMEGA-3

Don't pay too much attention to the total time in baking this bread. It truly is very easy and worth the wait. This recipe is great for making every one to two weeks. The large round of bread is wonderful for immediate, tomorrow, and later use. Enjoy the crisp warm exterior of the fresh bread. Divide a portion to be used over the next couple days. Slice and freeze individual slices that can be thawed and toasted over the next week or two. The basic recipe can work with all spelt flour or all white whole wheat, but I prefer the combination of the two. Have fun with different seed additions. Ground chia seed goes unnoticed and offers a boost of omega-3 fatty acids.

Ingredients:

3 c. spelt flour
3 c. white whole-wheat flour
3 tbsp. ground chia seeds
3½ c. warm water
1 tsp. dry yeast
1 tbsp. maple syrup
2½ to 3 tsp. salt

Directions:

In a large bowl combine the flours and chia seeds. In a separate bowl stir together the water, yeast, maple syrup, and salt until salt is dissolved. Add the wet mixture into the dry mixture creating wet dough. Place the dough on a well-floured surface and shape it into a large round piece of dough. Place the rounded dough in a lightly floured clean bowl. Cover the bowl with a clean towel and let sit to rise for about 8 hours or overnight.

Preheat the oven to 475 degrees. Place a cast-iron skillet in the oven to heat for about 15 minutes. Remove and very lightly flour the skillet. Place the dough in the skillet and cover with a lid. Bake for about 40 minutes. Remove the lid and reduce the temperature to 425 degrees. Bake for about 20 minutes, or until the bread makes a hollow sound when you knock on the center. Serve immediately or store for later use.

Nutrition per serving is approximately:

118 calories, 1 g fat, 225 to 325 mg sodium, 130 mg K, 25 g carbohydrate, 4 g fiber, 5 g protein, 0 percent vitamin A, 0 percent B12, 5 percent B6, 0 percent vitamin C, 0 percent vitamin D, 1 percent vitamin E, 2 percent calcium, 8 percent copper, 3 percent folate, 8 percent iron, 11 percent magnesium, 55 percent manganese, 11 percent niacin, 4 percent pantothenic acid, 13 percent phosphorus, 17 percent selenium, 8 percent thiamin, 7 percent zinc, 145 mg omega-3

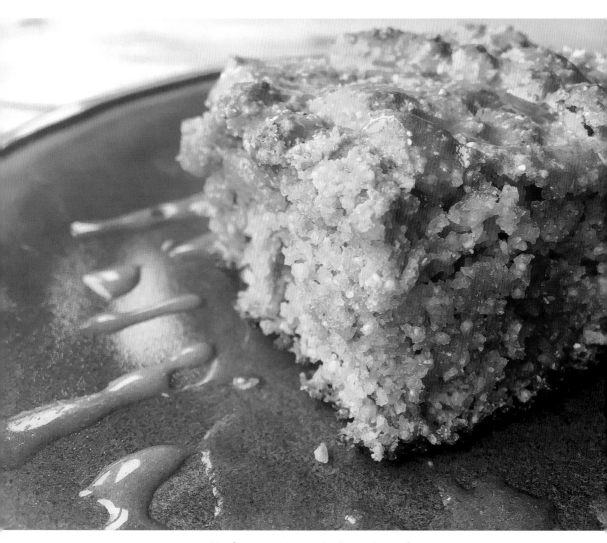

Endurance Lover's Corn Bread

Finish Line Fueling

Endurance Lover's Corn Bread

SERVES 9
TOTAL TIME: 40 MINUTES

VEGETARIAN, PRE-RACE, RECOVERY

There was a time when I was eating this corn bread recipe the day before marathons and as a pre-race meal to support stocking glycogen stores. The recipe offers a nice balance in terms of low fat, rich in carbohydrates, and moderate in protein. A couple pieces of corn bread with a good spread of honey about 90 to 120 minutes before race start provided me with a light, fueled, and race-ready feeling. Pair the meal with water or an electrolyte-containing beverage in effort to aim for light-colored urine.

Ingredients:

1 c. cornmeal
1 c. whole-wheat pastry flour
1 tsp. baking soda
1½ tsp. baking powder
¼ tsp. salt
¼ c. honey
1 c. pumpkin puree, canned or fresh
1 omega-3 large egg
¾ c. plain Greek yogurt
1 tbsp. extra virgin olive or high oleic safflower oil
¼ to ½ tsp. cinnamon (optional)

Directions:

Very lightly coat an 8 x 8-inch baking pan with a touch of extra virgin coconut oil. Preheat the oven to 375 degrees.

Combine all of the dry ingredients in a medium bowl. Add wet ingredients and mix by hand with a spoon until well blended. The batter will be fairly thick. Evenly spread the batter in the 8 x 8-inch baking pan.

Bake the corn bread batter for 30 minutes or until the top is lightly browned and the center is cooked with a very slight doughy appearance. Be careful not to overcook. Remove and cool slightly before serving.

Tip: Great served with cinnamon honey butter.

Nutrition per serving is approximately:

183 calories, 3 g fat, 52 mg potassium, 243 mg sodium, 35 g carbohydrates, 3.5 g fiber, 6 g protein, 130 percent vitamin A, 3 percent B12, 3 percent B6, 21 percent vitamin C, 0 percent vitamin D, 3 percent vitamin E, 9 percent calcium, 10 percent copper, 3 percent folate, 12 percent iron, 6 percent magnesium, 6 percent manganese, 3 percent niacin, 2 percent pantothenic acid, 7 percent phosphorus, 4 percent riboflavin, 3 percent selenium, 4 percent thiamin, 3 percent zinc

Long Run Toast

SERVES 1
TOTAL TIME: 5 MINUTES

VEGETARIAN, QUICK-TO-FIX, PRE-RUN, RECOVERY, MAGNESIUM PROBIOTICS, OMEGA-3

Many, many of my best runs were fueled by a simple toast breakfast or post-run snack. Pair a simple toast with a source of protein if the bread does not carry much protein. Greek or soy yogurt, hard-boiled egg, or a couple ounces of lean meat can offer just the right amount of protein to balance the basic pre-run or recovery meal.

Ingredients:

2 slices Chia Spelt Bread
2 tbsp. cinnamon honey butter
4 tbsp. yogurt

Directions:

Slice and toast the chia bread. Spread with honey butter, or use the fruit puree from the fruit on the bottom yogurt recipe. Top with a layer of yogurt.

Nutrition is approximately:

448 calories, 7 g fat, 530 to 730 mg sodium, 530 mg K, 94 g carbohydrate, 8 g fiber, 16 g protein, 5 percent vitamin A, 10 percent B12, 13 percent B6, 0 percent vitamin C, 0 percent vitamin D, 2 percent vitamin E, 12 percent calcium, 19 percent copper, 8 percent folate, 18 percent iron, 27 percent magnesium, 114 percent manganese, 22 percent niacin, 15 percent pantothenic acid, 42 percent phosphorus, 16 percent riboflavin, 44 percent selenium, 19 percent thiamin, 20 percent zinc, 290 mg omega-3

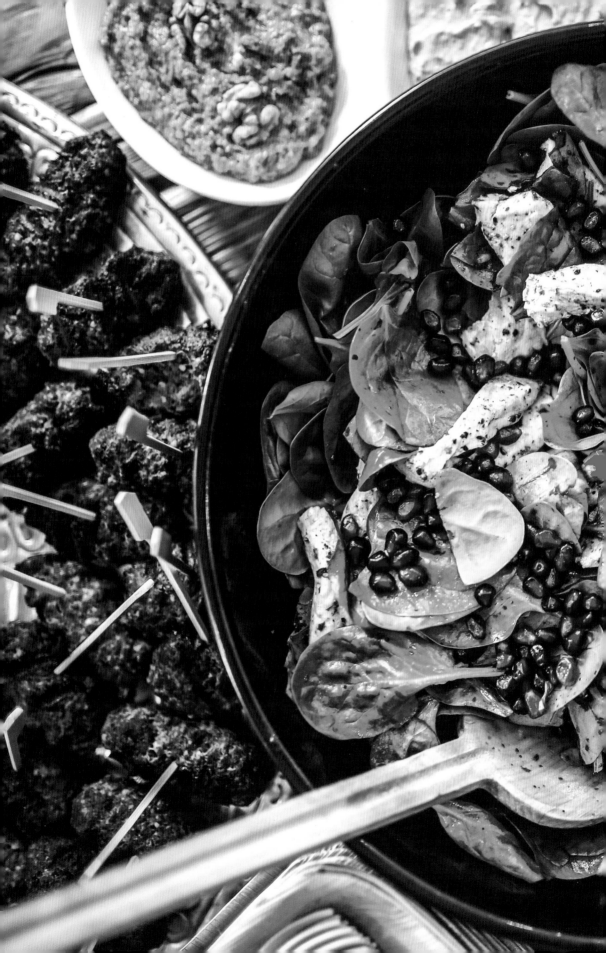

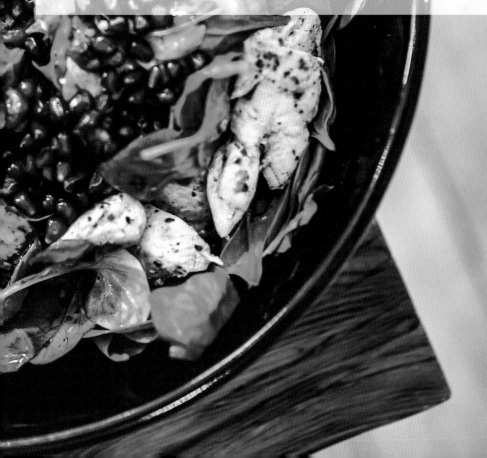

Salads and Soups

Nutrient-Packed Chopped Salad

SERVES 1
TOTAL TIME: 15 MINUTES

GLUTEN-FREE, B12, IRON, MAGNESIUM, VITAMIN D, QUICK-TO-FIX, HYDRATING

A large salad by itself may not be packed with glycogen-stocking carbohydrates, but it is still loaded with so many powerful nutrients. There are some days a heaping salad loaded with amazing ingredients is not only craved, but beneficial as part of a healthy diet. Salad dressing is not required with this fantastic nutrient boosting salad. The flavor from the olive, avocado, nutritional yeast, as well as the moisture drawn out from the salt offers a delicate pleasant flavor. Simply pair the salad base with a carbohydrate-rich side or topping such as fresh fruit, large sweet potato, whole grain crackers, bread, pasta, or brown rice to meet a fundamental fueling carbohydrate balance for the meal.

Ingredients:

2 c. spinach, chopped
2 c. romaine lettuce, chopped
⅓ cucumber, chopped
¼ medium tomato, chopped
8 jumbo black olives, sliced
¼ avocado, chopped
4 to 5 vitamin D mushrooms, chopped
3 oz. shredded cooked chicken breast
¼ tsp. salt
⅛ tsp. black pepper
1 tbsp. nutritional yeast

Directions:

In large bowl toss together all chopped vegetables and chicken. Add salt, pepper, and nutritional yeast and gently toss salad ingredients together. Transfer to serving bowl and serve.

Boil a fresh chicken breast for about 15 minutes if leftovers are not available.

Nutrition is approximately:

339 calories, 15 g fat, 1,119 mg potassium, 706.7 mg sodium, 25 g carbs, 10.5 g fiber, 31 g protein, 226 percent vitamin A, 86 percent vitamin C, 100 percent vitamin D, 46 percent B12, 183 percent B6, 20.6 percent vitamin E, 37 percent iron, 28 percent magnesium, 37.5 percent manganese, 140 percent niacin, 56 percent pantothenic acid, 194 percent riboflavin, 43 percent selenium, 196 percent thiamin, 21 percent zinc

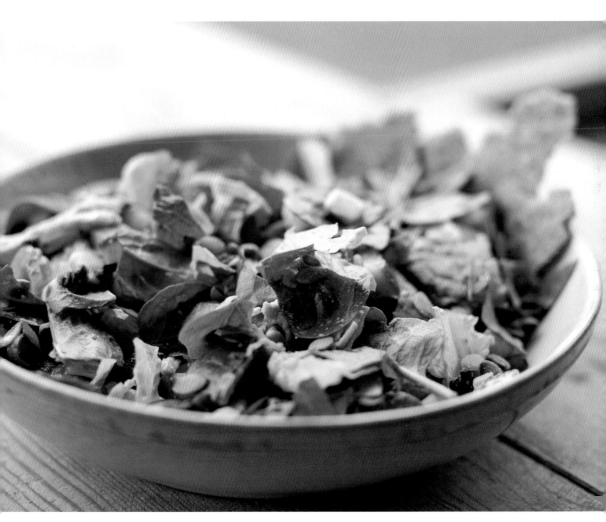

Nutrient-Packed Chopped Salad

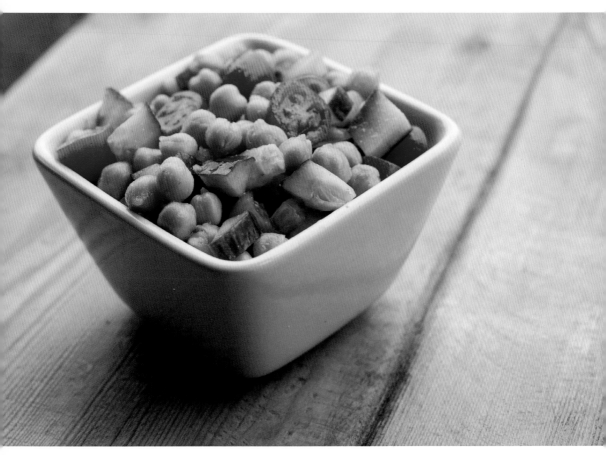

Seasoned Chickpea Salad

Seasoned Chickpea Salad

SERVES 2
TOTAL TIME: 35 MINUTES

VEGETARIAN, VEGAN, GLUTEN-FREE, QUICK-TO-FIX

Seasoned chickpeas with chopped vegetables can work great as a standalone meal, quick side dish, salad topping and even a flavor boosting pasta or soup ingredient. It's a fast, easy, and delicious go-to option for a runner pinched for time. Sprinkle chickpeas with nutritional yeast to offer a boost of B vitamins. Pair the meal with fresh fruit, toast, and cup of milk to round out this meal with additional carbohydrates and protein.

Ingredients:

½ tsp. garlic powder
½ tsp. onion powder
½ tsp. cumin
¼ to ½ tsp. salt (as desired)
1 tsp. olive oil
⅓ English cucumber, diced
¼ c. cherry tomatoes, halved
1½ c. cooked or canned chickpeas,
    rinsed and drained

Directions:

In a bowl combine garlic powder, onion powder, cumin, salt, and olive oil. Add the vegetables and beans and toss.

Nutrition per serving is approximately:

261 calories, 4 g fat, 803 mg sodium, 522 mg potassium, 47 g carbohydrate, 9 g fiber, 10 g protein, 18 percent vitamin A, 0 percent B12, 44 percent B6, 35 percent vitamin C, 7 percent calcium, 16 percent copper, 30 percent folate, 15 percent iron, 19 percent magnesium, 55 percent manganese, 6 percent niacin, 5 percent pantothenic acid, 17 percent phosphorus, 4 percent riboflavin, 8 percent selenium, 4 percent thiamin, 13 percent zinc

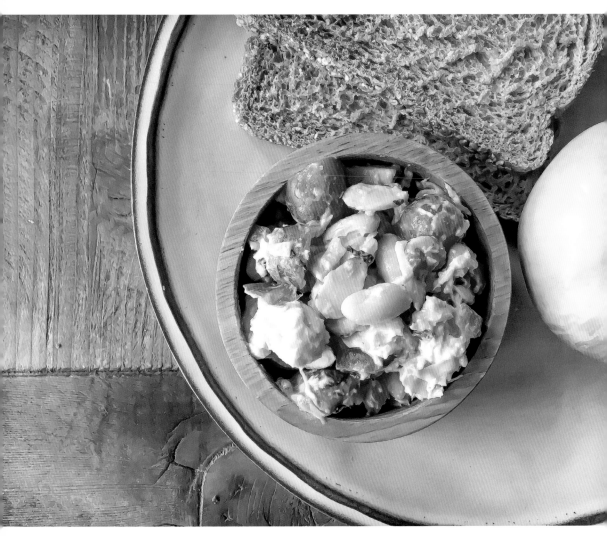

Chicken and White Bean Salad

Chicken and White Bean Salad

SERVES 4
TOTAL TIME: 35 MINUTES

QUICK-TO-FIX, B12, IRON, MAGNESIUM, PROBIOTICS

A boiled chicken breast recipe is a great opportunity to make extra shredded chicken to store for future meals. Pair the lean protein with colorful, antioxidant-rich fruits and vegetables. Chicken and white bean salad is delicious by itself, stuffed in a large leaf lettuce wrap, pita filling, or topped on toast. Balance the salad with carbohydrate-rich additions.

Ingredients:

2 c. boiled, chopped chicken breast
2 c. halved cherry tomatoes
½ c. chopped green onion
½ c. finely diced red bell pepper
1½ lemon, juiced
¾ c. plain grass-fed whole milk yogurt
1 15-oz. can white beans, rinsed
½ avocado, chopped
½–¾ tsp. salt
⅛ tsp. black pepper
1 packed tbsp. fresh basil, chopped
¼ c. slivered almonds

Directions:

Boil about 1 pound of raw chicken breast or chicken tenders in a medium saucepan for about 10 to 15 minutes until cooked through. Drain and chop the chicken. Toss the chicken in 1 tbsp. lemon juice and ¼ c. green onion. Set aside to cool.

Combine yogurt, salt, basil, pepper, and the rest of the green onion.

In a medium to large bowl combine the beans, red pepper, tomato, and cooled chicken breast. Toss with yogurt mixture. Gently fold in almonds and avocado. Best served after chilling for 20 to 30 minutes.

Nutrition per serving is approximately:

336 calories, 10 g fat, 582 mg sodium, 982 mg potassium, 42 g carbohydrate, 11 g fiber, 23 g protein, 32 percent vitamin A, 34 percent B12, 19 percent B6, 105 percent vitamin C, 0 percent vitamin D, 9 percent vitamin E, 21 percent calcium, 26 percent copper, 27 percent folate, 28 percent iron, 28 percent magnesium, 45 percent manganese, 25 percent niacin, 11 percent pantothenic acid, 29 percent phosphorus, 13 percent riboflavin, 15 percent selenium, 13 percent thiamin, 16 percent zinc

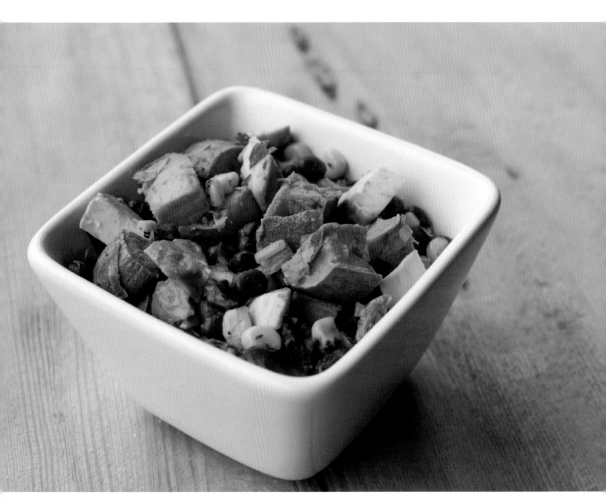

Southwest Sweet Potato Salad

Finish Line Fueling

Southwest Sweet Potato Salad

4 LARGE SERVINGS
TOTAL TIME: 35 MINUTES

VEGETARIAN, VEGAN, GLUTEN-FREE, MAGNESIUM

Southwest sweet potato salad was modified from a recipe I fell in love with years ago from "Two Peas and Their Pod." Instead of grilling the sweet potatoes I use roasted corn and bake the sweet potatoes.

Ingredients:

1 tbsp. extra virgin olive oil
¼ tsp. salt
3 sweet potatoes, cleaned and diced
1 can black beans, rinsed and drained
1 c. roasted frozen corn
½ c. cilantro
2 green onions, minced
2 fresh squeezed limes, or ¼ c. lime juice
2 ripe avocado, diced
Additional salt and pepper to taste

Directions:

Preheat oven to 425 degrees. Toss the olive oil, salt and sweet potato together. Bake the sweet potatoes on a cookie sheet for about 25 minutes until cooked through. Remove and set aside to cool.

In a large bowl combine the black beans, corn, cilantro, green onion, and half of the lime juice. Add the cooled sweet potato and toss to combine. Toss the avocado with the remaining lime juice and add mixture to the large bowl. Gently fold in the avocado, remaining lime juice, and any additional salt and pepper to taste. Serve right away or chill for about 1 hour before serving.

Tip: This recipe can serve as a meal or a side dish. If used as a meal, consider pairing the recipe with a couple ounces of lean chicken or beef, cup of milk, or nutritional yeast and extra beans to boost the protein and B12 content of the meal.

Nutrition per serving is approximately:

409 calories, 18 g fat, 173 mg sodium, 1,297 mg potassium, 57 g carbohydrate, 17.5 g fiber, 12.5 g protein, 110 percent vitamin A, 36 percent B6, 49 percent vitamin C, 7 percent calcium, 33 percent copper, 58 percent folate, 20 percent iron, 28 percent magnesium, 51 percent manganese, 22 percent niacin, 31 percent pantothenic acid, 28 percent phosphorus, 20 percent riboflavin, 4 percent selenium, 30 percent thiamin, 15 percent zinc

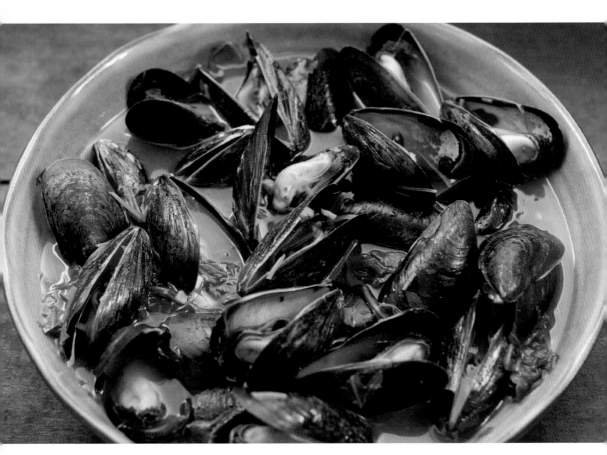

Herb Mussels

Herb Mussels

SERVES 2
TOTAL TIME: 35 MINUTES

VEGETARIAN, GLUTEN-FREE, B12, IRON, OMEGA-3, QUICK-TO-FIX, HYDRATING, RECOVERY

Shellfish such as mussels, oysters, and clams are an excellent source of nutrition for a heavy training runner. They can serve a major role in meeting a runner's B12, iron, selenium, zinc, omega-3 fatty acids, and iodine needs, among other great nutrients. Not only are mussels one of the fastest meals to be made, the powerful dish will support a runner's immune system, thyroid function, and oxygen delivery. Pair this dish with quality carbohydrates such as brown rice, sweet potato, fruit, and fresh bread to meet recovery needs.

Ingredients:

1 lb. mussels, washed
2 c. seafood stock (chicken or vegetable broth can substitute)
2 cloves garlic, minced
1 tbsp. unsalted butter
½ tsp. thyme
1 c. loosely chopped baby arugula
Salt and pepper to taste

Directions:

In a large pot or skillet over medium heat, add butter and garlic. After about 1 to 2 minutes add the seafood stock, arugula, and thyme. Once the stock comes to a boil add the mussels and cover. After several minutes the mussels will begin to open. Once the mussels open remove from the heat immediately and serve. Discard any mussels that did not open. Add salt and pepper to taste.

Nutrition per serving is approximately:

270 calories, 11 g fat, 394 mg sodium, 429 mg potassium 16 g carbohydrate, 2 g fiber, 26 g protein, 28 percent vitamin A, 338 percent B12, 397 percent B6, 12 percent B6, 38 percent vitamin C, 2 percent vitamin D, 2 percent vitamin E, 11 percent calcium, 12 percent copper, 25 percent folate, 44 percent iron, 12 percent magnesium, 349 percent manganese, 18 percent niacin, 12 percent pantothenic acid, 32 percent phosphorus, 28 percent riboflavin, 129 percent selenium, 46 percent thiamin, 20 percent zinc, 1125 mg omega-3

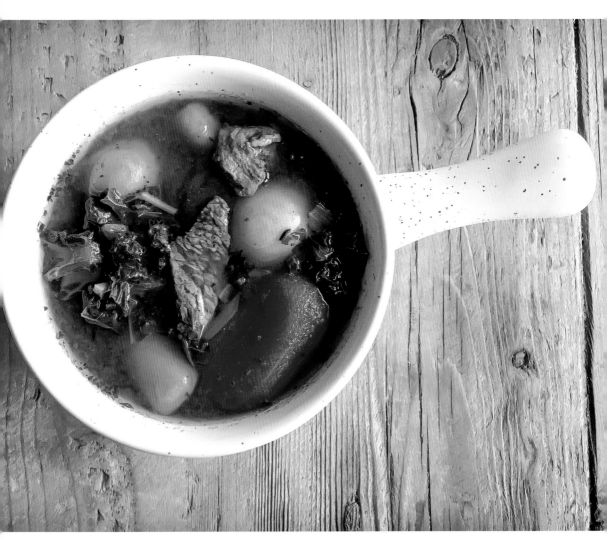

Basic Beef Stew

Basic Beef Stew

SERVES 6
TOTAL TIME: 8 HOURS + 15 MINUTES

GLUTEN-FREE, IRON, B12, HYDRATING, RECOVERY

Making a basic beef stew reminds me of stuffing a gym bag quickly in the morning before running out the door. Since there is very little need to cut and peel, this is so fast and convenient. It offers as a winter warmer after a cold hard effort, and supports rehydration after a summer dehydrating workout. Pair a bowl of beef stew with fresh bread, fruit, a side of brown rice or buttered noodles to meet carbohydrate needs.

Ingredients:

1 package or 16 oz. beef stew meat
1 tsp. extra virgin olive oil
½ large white onion
½ tsp. + 1 tsp. salt
½ tsp. + ½ tsp. dried thyme
½ tsp. + ½ tsp. dried sage
2 to 3 cloves garlic, minced
1 bag white new potatoes
1 12-oz. bag carrots
1 16-oz. bag frozen kale
1 18-oz. jar stewed whole tomatoes
2 bay leaves
54 ounces water

Directions:

In a medium to large skillet over medium heat combine stew meat, olive oil, onion, ½ tsp. salt, ½ tsp. thyme, and ½ tsp. sage and cook until the stew meat is just brown on the outside.

In a large crockpot combine all of the ingredients and cook for 8 hours. Serve warm.

Nutrition per serving is approximately:

465 calories, 15 g fat, 57 g carb, 4.5 g fiber, 23 g protein, 882 mg sodium, 632 mg potassium, 113 percent vitamin A, 30 percent B12, 15 percent B6, 76 percent vitamin C, 0 percent vitamin D, 2 percent vitamin E, 13 percent calcium, 6 percent copper, 2 percent folate, 28 percent iron, 3 percent magnesium, 4 percent manganese, 17 percent niacin, 1 percent pantothenic acid, 2 percent phosphorus, 9 percent riboflavin, 1 percent selenium, 3 percent thiamin, 18 percent zinc

Butternut Apple Soup

SERVES 6
TOTAL TIME: 75 MINUTES

VEGETARAN, VEGAN, GLUTEN-FREE, PRE-RUN, POST-RUN, HYDRATING

Coming home from a run to the smell of fresh baked squash is wonderful. Before heading out the door for a late day run place a butternut squash in a warm oven. It's a great way to get dinner started while working in a run for the day. Squash is a forgiving, oven-friendly cooking option if a great workout warrants a couple more miles.

This soup alone lacks the balance a full meal requires. Apple butternut soup works great paired with grilled lean steak, bison burger, or other iron-rich protein sources. The vitamin C in the recipe and lack of calcium supports iron absorption. The soup supports hydration before a warm summer run or after a high sweat loss workout.

Roasted polenta, fresh fruit, or a whole grain baguette can supply carbohydrate to replenish glycogen stores. Ginger root offers a pleasant flavor and anti-inflammatory boost to mealtime. Store and use any leftovers as a future pasta sauce or a seasoning for beans and rice.

Ingredients:

1 large butternut squash (yield about
    4 c. butternut cooked)
2 apples, chopped with skins
32 oz. vegetable broth
1 tbsp. extra virgin olive oil
1 tbsp. fresh minced ginger root
¼ tsp. ground sage
¼ tsp. ground nutmeg
¼ c. culinary coconut milk
½ to 1 c. low fat milk, unsweetened
    almond, or coconut milk (optional)

Toppings:

Pumpkin seeds or walnuts (optional)
Greek yogurt (optional)

Directions:

Preheat oven to 400 degrees. Cut the butternut squash in half. It helps to first cut off the stem. Place each half face down on a parchment paper–lined cookie sheet and bake for about 1 hour until soft.

When the squash is fully cooked remove it from the oven. Discard the seeds and scoop out the soft butternut squash with a spoon. It should produce about 4 cups of cooked squash.

In a large pot over medium heat combine the ginger, apples, olive oil, sage, and nutmeg, cooking the apples down until soft. Add the squash and vegetable broth. Once the soup warms to a near slow boil, turn off the heat, and blend the soup with an immersion blender until smooth. Fold in the coconut milk and serve. For a thinner consistency add ½ to 1 c. of milk as desired.

Nutrition per serving is approximately:

120 calories, 3.5 g fat, 944 mg sodium, 57 mg potassium, 22 g carbohydrate, 3.5 g fiber, 1 g protein, 234 percent vitamin A, 0 percent B12, 10 percent B6, 41 percent vitamin C, 0 percent vitamin D, 3 percent vitamin E, 6 percent calcium, 5 percent copper, 0.5 percent folate, 6 percent iron, 10 percent magnesium, 1 percent manganese, 6 percent niacin, 5 percent pantothenic acid, 4 percent phosphorus, 2 percent riboflavin, 0.2 percent selenium, 7 percent thiamin, 1 percent zinc

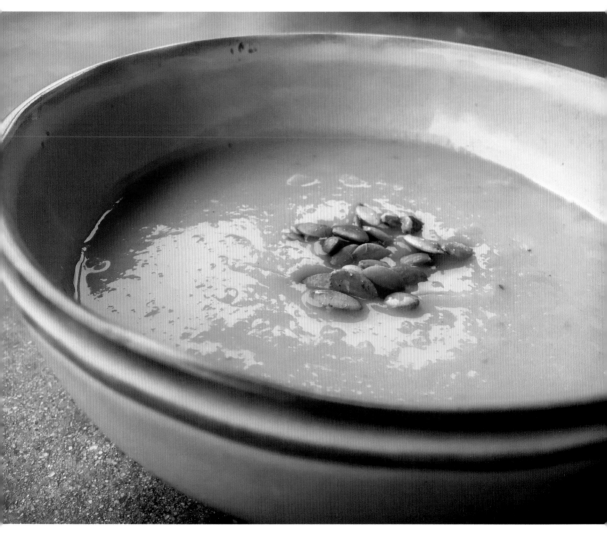

Butternut Apple Soup

Root Soup

VEGETARIAN, VEGAN, GLUTEN-FREE, IRON, CALCIUM MAGNESIUM, HYDRATING

Root soup is a favorite way to work in beets and a fantastic assortment of anti-inflammatory ingredients. A large helping served with fresh fruit and warm bread can make a meal. A smaller serving can complement a sandwich or salad. Pair this with post-run fueling to support recovery and hydration.

Ingredients:

1 tsp. olive oil
¼ c. minced turmeric root
1 small onion, chopped (about 1 c.)
2 beets, chopped into small pieces (about 2 c.)
1 small turnip, chopped into small pieces (about 1 c.)
1 rutabaga, chopped into small pieces (about 1 c.)
2 carrots, chopped
32 oz. chicken or vegetable broth
1 tbsp. minced ginger root
1 c. low fat milk (1 percent) or coconut or almond milk

Toppings:

1 c. whole milk grass-fed yogurt
fresh dill, or other fresh herb (optional)

Directions:

In a large pot over medium heat combine the olive oil, turmeric, onion, beets, turnip, rutabaga, and carrots. Cover with a lid and cook, occasionally stirring, for about 10 minutes. Add the broth and bring it to a slow boil. Cover and cook for about 20 minutes, until the beets and other vegetables are soft.

Add the ginger. With an immersion or stick blender, puree the soup until smooth. As it begins to thicken add the milk, again blending until smooth. Add any additional salt to taste.

Serve with yogurt and sprinkle of fresh dill, or any fresh herbs on hand.

Tip: Consider purchasing organic vegetables and washing them well. Skip vegetable peeling to save time and offer the nutrition present in the skin. The only exception in this recipe is to peel the skin layer of the ginger. Always chop vegetables the same size for even cooking.

Makes approximately 6½ to 7 cups.

Nutrition per serving is approximately:

191 calories, 5 g fat, 1,168 mg sodium, 1,446 mg potassium, 28 g carbohydrate, 4 g fiber, 10 g protein, 97 percent vitamin A, 22 percent B12, 12 percent B6, 35 percent vitamin C, 16 percent

vitamin D, 4 percent vitamin E, 27 percent calcium, 19 percent copper, 14 percent folate, 26 percent iron, 15 percent magnesium, 38 percent manganese, 33 percent niacin, 10 percent pantothenic acid, 37 percent phosphorus, 28 percent riboflavin, 17 percent selenium, 7 percent thiamin, 12 percent zinc

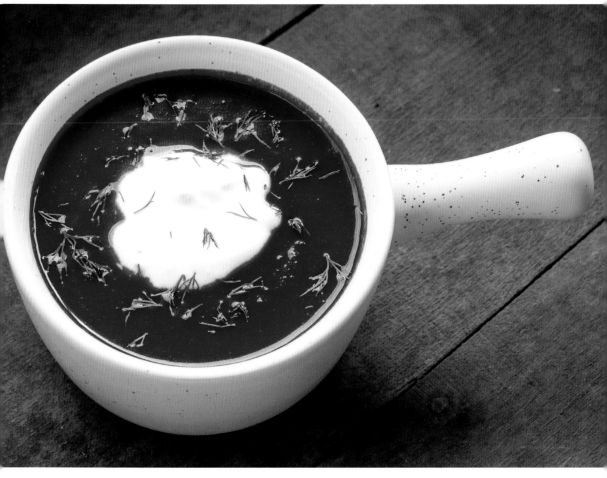

Root Soup

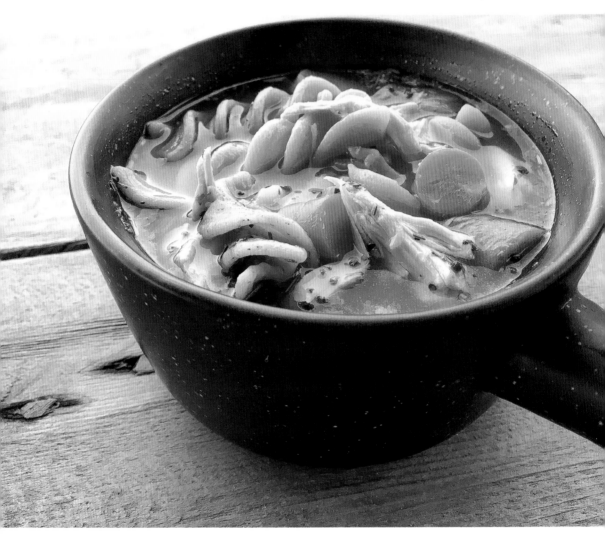

Chicken Noodle Soup

Finish Line Fueling

Chicken Noodle Soup

SERVES 4
TOTAL TIME: 40 MINUTES

PRE-RUN, POST-RUN, HYDRATING

As a working mom at the peak of training 80 to 100 miles a week, there are days I wanted a meal fast, but with fresh from home quality. Meals can come together quickly and budget friendly with a quick visit to a natural foods store for sale rotisserie day. Pick up a plain organic rotisserie chicken. It can be a big help in making a hearty meal like a chicken noodle soup in no time.

Ingredients:

16 oz. package of pasta noodles, high fiber
1 tbsp. extra virgin olive oil
3 c. sliced carrots
1 c. chopped onion
32 oz. chicken broth
1 tsp. dried thyme
1 tsp. dried marjoram
1 plain organic rotisserie chicken, cooked and meat removed from the bone
2 to 3 c. cooking water from cooked noodles

Directions:

Cook pasta noodles according to directions.

In a large pot over medium heat combine the oil, carrot, and onion. Cover the pot and let the vegetables cook, stirring occasionally, until nearly soft. Add the chicken broth, thyme, marjoram, and rotisserie chicken. Cover and bring to a slow simmer for about 5 minutes.

Add about 5 c. pasta noodles and 3 c. of the starchy water remaining from the cooked noodles. Season the soup with any additional salt and pepper to taste.

Reserve leftover pasta noodles for a future meal.

Nutrition is approximately:

425 calories, 6 g fat, 65 g carb, 9 g fiber, 31 g protein, 958 mg sodium, 752 mg potassium, 159 percent vitamin A, 14 percent B12, 18 percent B6, 9 percent vitamin C, 0 percent vitamin D, 4 percent calcium, 11 percent copper, 9 percent folate, 35 percent iron, 7 percent magnesium, 23 percent manganese, 36 percent niacin, 3 percent pantothenic acid, 32 percent phosphorus, 7 percent riboflavin, 40 percent selenium, 4 percent thiamin, 8 percent zinc

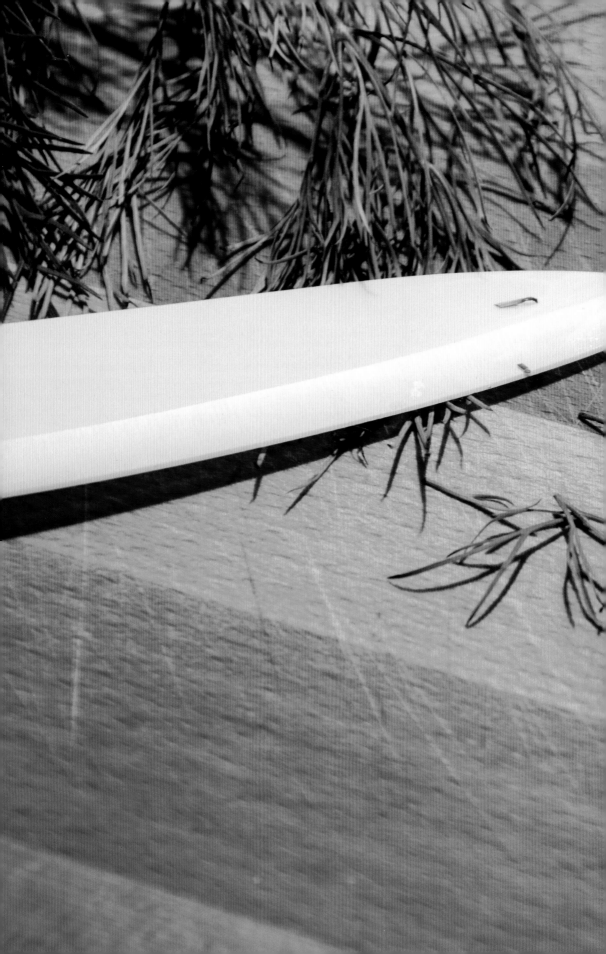

Main Dishes

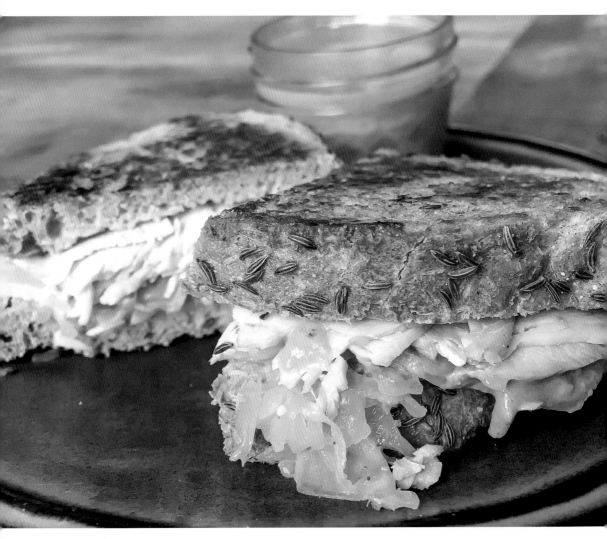

Turkey Reuben

Turkey Reuben

SERVES 1
TOTAL TIME: 15 MINUTES

PRE-RUN, POST-RUN, QUICK-TO-FIX, B12, PROBIOTICS

This quick meal offers as a great source of immune system supporting probiotics. Probiotics can be killed during heating, but the probiotics in this sandwich are preserved nicely in the sandwich. Enjoy the sandwich with fresh fruit, milk, or Medjool dates to boost the carbohydrate content of the meal.

Ingredients:

2 slices fresh bakery rye bread
3 ounces shaved turkey breast
1 slice Swiss cheese
2 to 3 heaping tbsp. sauerkraut
2 tbsp. plain grass-fed whole milk
    yogurt
2 tbsp. ketchup
½ tsp. horseradish
olive oil, to taste

Directions:

In a small bowl combine the yogurt, ketchup, and horseradish and set aside.

In a skillet over medium heat drizzle the olive oil. Gently spread one side of each slice of bread across the warm olive oil to lightly coat. Remove the bread. Layer the toppings on one slice of bread, on the side not coated in olive oil. Begin with the slice of cheese followed by the yogurt dressing, sauerkraut, and turkey. Top with the other slice of bread, olive oil side facing out. Toast the bread on the skillet for about 3 to 5 minutes each side until the bread is toasted and the cheese begins to melt. Serve immediately.

Nutrition is approximately:

435 calories, 15 g fat, 44 g carb, 4 g fiber, 28 g protein, 1,089 mg sodium, 319 mg potassium, 10 percent vitamin A, 30 percent B12, 20 percent B6, 13 percent vitamin C, 3 percent vitamin D, 37 percent calcium, 9 percent copper, 16 percent folate, 17 percent iron, 14 percent magnesium, 28 percent manganese, 13 percent niacin, 10 percent pantothenic acid, 47 percent phosphorus, 37 percent riboflavin, 72 percent selenium, 27 percent thiamin, 20 percent zinc

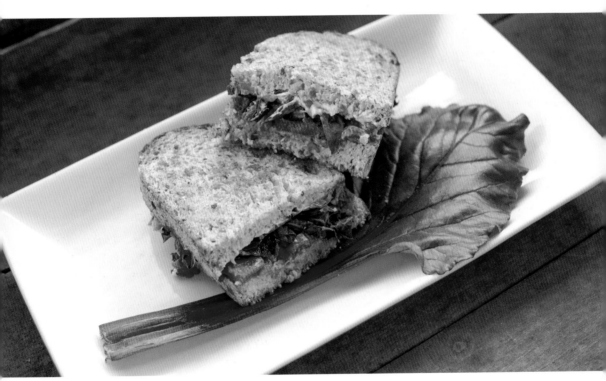

Rainbow Goat Basil Sandwich

Finish Line Fueling

Rainbow Goat Basil Sandwich

SERVES 1
TOTAL TIME: 15 MINUTES

VEGETARIAN, PRE-RUN, POST-RUN, QUICK-TO-FIX

Have you ever noticed a state of discontent after eating a meal of only cold items? Instead of searching the cabinets to fill the void later, consider incorporating warm items into meal-time. The same sandwich meal, yet warm, may provide the satisfaction needed. This savory warm sandwich is delicious any time of day, including before a demanding workout. Pair the sandwich with fruit, low fat milk, soup, crackers, yogurt, or even a sweet potato to meet your target carbohydrate range.

Ingredients:

2 slices bakery fresh whole grain bread
2 tbsp. goat cheese log
1 tbsp. chives
1 rainbow chard leaf, chopped
1 tbsp. balsamic vinegar
¼ c. fresh or from a jar roasted red pepper
1 tbsp. loosely chopped basil
½ tsp. olive oil

Directions:

In a small bowl combine goat cheese and chives.

In a skillet over medium heat drizzle the olive oil. Gently spread one side of each slice of bread across the olive oil to lightly coat. Remove the bread.

Sauté the chard with balsamic vinegar until the chard softens. Layer the toppings on one slice of bread on the side not coated in olive oil. Begin with the goat cheese followed by the chard, red pepper, and basil.

Top with the other slice of bread, olive oil side facing out. Toast the bread on the skillet for about 3 to 5 minutes each side, until the bread is toasted and the cheese begins to melt. Serve immediately.

Nutrition is approximately:

472 calories, 11 g fat, 700 mg sodium, 212 mg potassium, 50 g carbohydrate, 5 g fiber, 15 g protein, 76 percent vitamin A, 2 percent B12, 10 percent B6, 81 percent vitamin C, 0 percent vitamin D, 14 percent calcium, 13 percent copper, 24 percent folate, 19 percent iron, 10 percent magnesium, 9 percent manganese, 13 percent niacin, 3 percent pantothenic acid, 7 percent phosphorus, 16 percent riboflavin, 2 percent selenium, 22 percent thiamin, 3 percent zinc

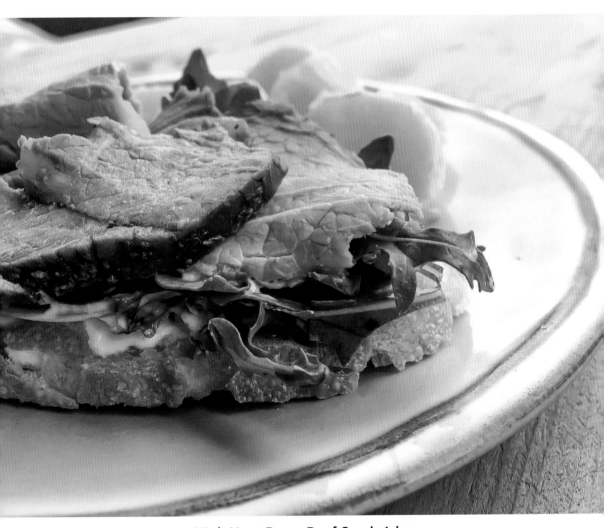

High Heat Roast Beef Sandwiches

Finish Line Fueling

High Heat Roast Beef Sandwiches

SERVES 4
TOTAL TIME: 75 MINUTES

B12, IRON, PROBIOTICS

Make a quick beef meal easy and worry-free. Place the prepped roast beef in the oven. Slip on your running gear and turn the oven off. Return from your run to the delicious smell of a wonderful, low maintenance meal. Working in a beef dish such as high heat roast beef 1 to 2 meals a week supports B12, iron, and zinc intake, which are all critical nutrients for a runner. Combine this meal with clementine, fresh berries, or grapefruit to boost the carbohydrate and vitamin C content. Pair vitamin C-containing foods with high iron foods to support iron absorption.

Ingredients:

½ tsp. sage
½ tsp. thyme
½ tsp. salt
½ tsp. garlic powder
1 lb. eye of round roast beef

Horseradish Cream:

¼ c. low fat grass-fed sour cream (or whole milk yogurt)
1 tsp. horseradish
1 tsp. lemon juice
salt and pepper to taste

Bring it Together:

Large-slice sourdough or whole grain bread
¼ c. arugula per sandwich

Directions:

Preheat the oven to 500 degrees. Combine sage, thyme, salt, and garlic powder in a small bowl. Rub the dry spice mixture to coat the entire roast. Place the roast in a shallow baking dish and place in the oven, uncovered. Cook the roast for 5 to 6 minutes per pound of meat for medium-well roast. Then turn off the oven. Do not open the oven for about 2 hours.

In a small bowl combine all of the horseradish cream toppings.

Toast bread and top with horseradish cream, arugula, and beef. Serve immediately.

Nutrition per sandwich is approximately:

517 calories, 15 g fat, 51 g carb, 3 g fiber, 41 g protein, 770 mg sodium, 412 mg potassium, 4 percent vitamin A, 72 percent B12, 23 percent B6, 5 percent vitamin C, 5 percent calcium, 0 percent vitamin D, 3 percent vitamin E, 14 percent copper, 40 percent folate, 28 percent iron, 13 percent magnesium, 26 percent manganese, 50 percent niacin, 11 percent pantothenic acid, 32 percent phosphorus, 30 percent riboflavin, 89 percent selenium, 39 percent thiamin, 42 percent zinc

Potatoes

Versatile is an excellent way to describe the potato. It can be baked, mashed, roasted, or turned into a bright colored, satisfying soup. It is a delicious source of fuel for any time of day—breakfast, lunch, or dinner. Top a sweet potato with cinnamon and almond butter for a quick breakfast, or season and roast it for a savory dinner meal. There's no need to reserve this delicious root vegetable for restaurant-style French fries or as a sugarcoated side at the annual Thanksgiving feast.

Incorporating potatoes offers a fantastic source of fuel for endurance athletes. The sweet potato contains glycogen-stocking carbohydrates to support energy needs for long, hard, or intense efforts. They offer nutrients such as vitamin A and C, beta-carotene, potassium, manganese, pantothenic acid, and fiber. The brilliant sweet potato color not only adds appeal to any dinner plate, it's a reminder that the sweet potato houses powerful anti-inflammatory phytonutrients.

Make It Quick-To-Fix:

Plan ahead by baking a batch of sweet potatoes all at once to dine on throughout the week.

- Slice or chop the sweet potato into smaller pieces for shorter cooking time. This is a great strategy for soups, roasted potatoes, and mashed potatoes.
- Prick the potato all over with a fork and microwave it for 8 to 10 minutes, until tender, turning the potato once.
- Half-baked–prick the potato with a fork and microwave for 3 to 5 minutes. Finish off the potato in the oven at 400 degrees for about 8 to 10 minutes, until tender, to get that fresh out of the oven flavor.
- Cut the sweet potato into ½ to 1-inch slices or wedges, season, and bake at 400 degrees for about 20 to 25 minutes.

All-In-One Stuffed Potato Meal Ingredients:

- Taco meat, black beans, salsa, cheddar cheese, plain Greek yogurt
- Avocado, salsa, chickpeas
- Black beans, arugula, and poached egg
- Cinnamon, coconut oil, plain Greek yogurt, and pumpkin seeds
- Feta cheese, olives, and sun-dried tomato
- Leftover chili and sharp cheddar cheese
- Additional delicious stuffing ingredients: lime juice, cilantro, chives, shredded chicken, corn, hemp seeds, green leafy vegetables, quinoa, brown or wild rice, broccoli, Brussels sprouts, and goat cheese

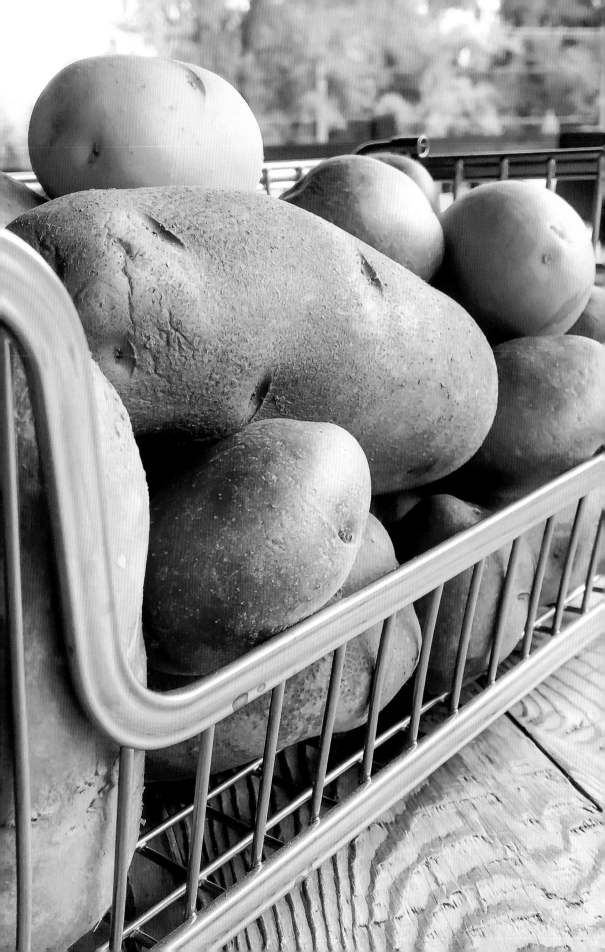

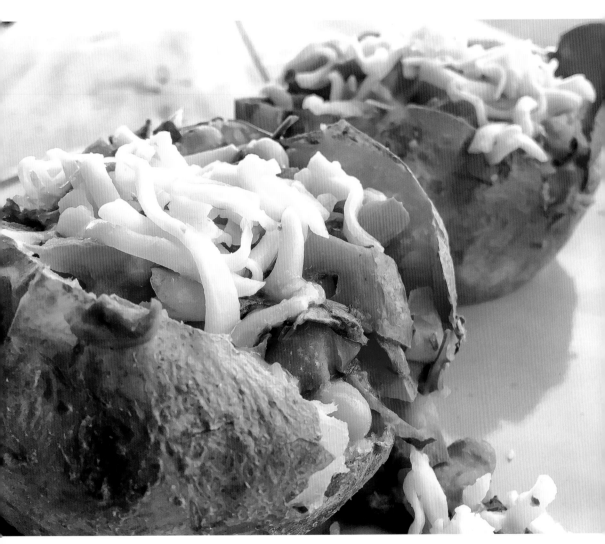

Stuffed Bean Potato

Finish Line Fueling

Stuffed Bean Potatoes

SERVES 4
TOTAL TIME: 75 MINUTES

VEGETARIAN, VEGAN, GLUTEN-FREE, IRON, VITAMIN D, MAGNESIUM, PROBIOTIC

Ingredients:

4 large potatoes, russet or sweet, washed and poked with a fork
1 red bell pepper, chopped
1 c. finely chopped vitamin D mushrooms
1 tbsp. avocado oil
2 cloves garlic, minced
2 c. loosely chopped arugula
1 large tomato, diced
1 can white beans, rinsed and drained
1 can kidney beans, rinsed and drained
1½ tsp. cumin
1 tsp. chili powder
1 to 1½ tsp. salt

Optional Toppings:

½ c. shredded pepper jack cheese (optional)
Plain grass-fed whole milk yogurt (optional)

Directions:

Preheat oven to 450 degrees. Place the potatoes on a baking sheet and bake for 60 to 70 minutes, until soft. (It's the perfect time to head out for a late run!)

When the potatoes are cooked through, combine the bell pepper, mushrooms, avocado oil, and garlic in a large skillet over medium heat. Cook until the bell pepper begins to soften. Add the arugula and tomatoes, cooking for another 3 to 5 minutes, until tomato softens and the arugula begins to wilt. Add the beans and spices. Cover and simmer on low for about 3 to 5 minutes.

Cut the potato halfway through. Gently mash the potato within the skin. Fill the potato with the warm bean mixture and top with cheese and yogurt.

Tip: A vegan athlete may want to consider nutritional yeast as a cheese-like topping to boost their daily B12 intake. Grass-fed whole milk yogurt will boost B12 and calcium for non-vegans.

Nutrition per stuffed potato (without cheese and yogurt) is approximately:

480 calories, 5 g fat, 91 g carbohydrates, 22 g fiber, 21 g protein, 1,046 mg sodium, 2,017 mg potassium, 238 percent vitamin A, 1 percent B12, 45 percent B6, 122 percent vitamin C, 56 percent vitamin D, 21 percent calcium, 10 percent vitamin E, 62 percent copper, 45 percent folate, 45 percent iron, 35 percent magnesium, 101 percent manganese, 27 percent niacin, 41 percent pantothenic acid, 43 percent phosphorus, 32 percent riboflavin, 10 percent selenium, 38 percent thiamin, 22 percent zinc

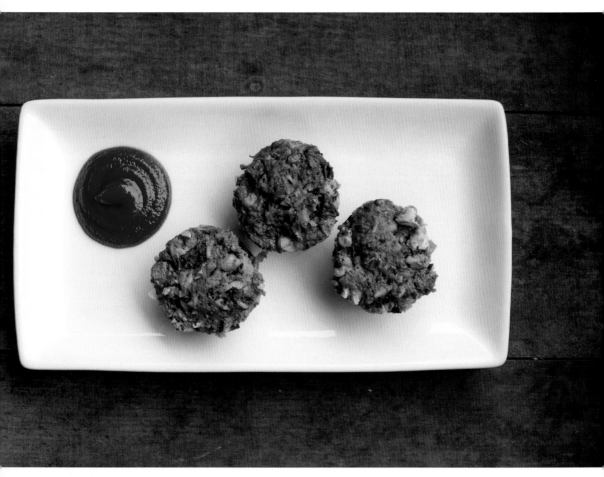

All-in-One Meatloaf Muffins

All-in-One Meatloaf Muffins

SERVES 12
TOTAL TIME: 30 MINUTES

GLUTEN-FREE, QUICK-TO-FIX, PRE-RUN, RECOVERY, B12, IRON, VITAMIN D

By baking the meatloaf in a muffin pan, this recipe is finished in no time. Another benefit of using the muffin pan is the perfectly sized portions that can be stored in the refrigerator or freezer for future use. Complement this meaty muffin with vitamin C rich fruit to boost iron absorption, as well as the carbohydrate content of the meal.

Serve meatloaf muffins with mashed or boiled potato, fresh bread, a cup of pasta, or a cup of peas to offer the additional necessary carbohydrate to fuel great training. Turn any leftovers into a sandwich for lunch the following day.

Ingredients:

16-oz. 90 percent lean bison, ground
1 can white beans
1 c. grated carrot, or 1 large grated carrot
1 c. finely chopped vitamin D mushrooms
⅔ c. brown rice, cooked
¼ c. chopped basil
1 tsp. thyme
1 egg
1 tsp. salt
1 to 2 garlic cloves, minced

Directions:

Preheat the oven to 350 degrees. Combine all ingredients in a medium-size bowl. Fill 12 muffin pan wells with meat mixture. Bake in the oven for about 20 to 22 minutes. Serve with ketchup, horseradish cream, or tzatziki.

Nutrition per 2 muffins is approximately:

269 calories, 12 g fat, 17 g carbohydrates, 3 g fiber, 27 g protein, 434 mg sodium, 581 mg potassium, 46 percent vitamin A, 29 percent B12, 20 percent B6, 3 percent vitamin C, 33 percent vitamin D, 10 percent calcium, 1 percent vitamin E, 20 percent copper, 22 percent folate, 32 percent iron, 21 percent magnesium, 41 percent manganese, 24 percent niacin, 12 percent pantothenic acid, 28 percent phosphorus, 15 percent riboflavin, 38 percent selenium, 16 percent thiamin, 35 percent zinc

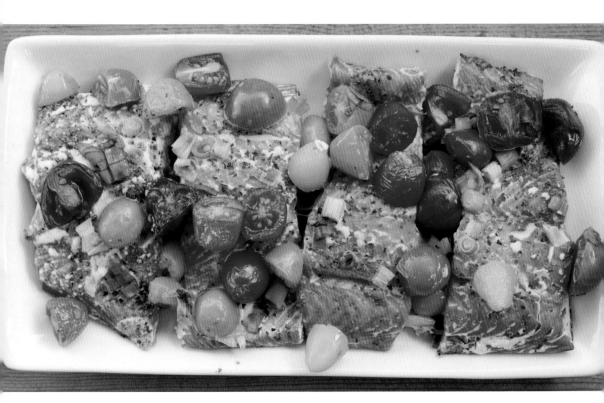

Salmon Steaks

Finish Line Fueling

Salmon Steaks

SERVES 4
TOTAL TIME: 30 MINUTES

VEGETARIAN, GLUTEN-FREE, QUICK-TO-FIX, B12, OMEGA-3

Salmon is a great fatty fish to support acquiring the anti-inflammatory benefits of omega-3 fatty acids. Salmon is also an excellent source of B12, protein, and iodine. Pair a salmon steak with spinach and mushrooms, wild rice, and fresh fruit to support meeting carbohydrate goals.

Ingredients:

1 lb. wild caught salmon, cut into 4
    sections
1 c. cherry tomatoes, halved
2 green onions
½ tsp. dried basil
¼ tsp. salt

Directions:

Preheat the oven to 425 degrees. Place salmon steaks on a parchment paper-lined baking sheet. Top the salmon with basil, salt, green onions, and tomatoes. Bake the salmon for about 15 to 18 minutes, or until the salmon steak reaches an internal temperature of 130 degrees. Let the salmon rest for about 5 minutes before serving.

Nutrition per steak is approximately:

251 calories, 11 g fat, 2 g carb, 1 g fiber, 34 g protein, 208 mg sodium, 844 mg potassium, 13 percent vitamin A, 86 percent B12, 81 percent B6, 13 percent vitamin C, 4 percent calcium, 0 percent vitamin D, 0 percent vitamin E, 4 percent calcium, 27 percent copper, 13 percent folate, 12 percent iron, 16 percent magnesium, 2 percent manganese, 85 percent niacin, 33 percent pantothenic acid, 44 percent phosphorus, 49 percent riboflavin, 114 percent selenium, 31 percent thiamin, 10 percent zinc, 4,396 mg omega-3

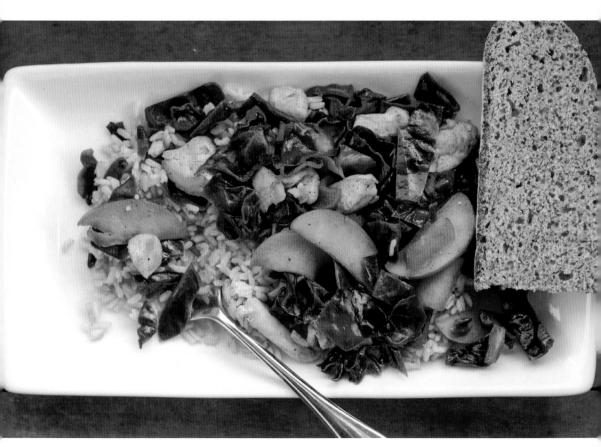

Chicken Apple Cabbage

Chicken Apple Cabbage

SERVES 4
TOTAL TIME: 40 MINUTES

GLUTEN-FREE, PRE-RUN, RECOVERY

Chicken apple cabbage is a great meal any time of day. The warm nutmeg flavor in the leftovers makes a very satisfying breakfast. Runners suffering from iron deficiency can pair this meal with an iron supplement, as the high vitamin C content supports iron absorption.

Ingredients:

5 c. or 1 small red cabbage, chopped
2 c. or 2 to 3 apples, thinly sliced
3 tbsp. unsalted butter
¼ + ¼ tsp. nutmeg, divided
⅛ tsp. black pepper
¼ + ¼ tsp. salt, divided
4 c. cooked brown rice
1 large chicken breast (about 12 ounces), diced
1 clove garlic, minced

Directions:

Prepare brown rice according to package directions.

In a large skillet, melt 2 tbsp. butter over medium heat. Add the cabbage, apples, black pepper, ¼ tsp. salt, and ¼ tsp. nutmeg. Sauté until cabbage and apples soften.

Preheat a separate small skillet or griddle to medium heat. Gently slide the tablespoon of butter over the pan or griddle to create a slight coating of butter in the pan. Remove the rest of the butter and set aside. Cook the chicken breast in the skillet with the garlic until fully cooked. Combine the garlic chicken with the apple cabbage in the large skillet.

Toss the remaining butter, nutmeg, and salt with the brown rice until combined. Top the brown rice with the chicken apple cabbage and serve.

Nutrition per serving is approximately:

460 calories, 13 g fat, 343 mg sodium, 643 mg potassium, 61 g carbohydrate, 7 g fiber, 26 g protein, 32 percent vitamin A, 6 percent B12, 36 percent B6, 113 percent vitamin C, 4 percent copper, 3 percent vitamin E, 11 percent iron, 7 percent calcium, 11 percent magnesium, 16 percent manganese, 50 percent niacin, 9 percent pantothenic acid, 10 percent riboflavin, 23 percent selenium, 10 percent thiamin, 6 percent zinc

Pumpkin Chili

SERVES 5
TOTAL TIME: 30 MINUTES

QUICK-TO-FIX, B12, IRON, MAGNESIUM

Ditch the pre-made chili-seasoning packet and create a flavorful chili with staple season-ings from the pantry. Be creative with vegetables and load the chili with vegetables rich in antioxidants. A warm chili is great for after a cold winter run or dehydrating, high sweat loss effort. Growing up in Cincinnati, I was raised with chili over noodles. This meal is a great way to boost the carbohydrate intake of the meal for a runner. Chili makes a wonderful top-ping on many carbohydrate-rich options like noodles, rice, potatoes, and quinoa.

Ingredients:

1 lb. 93 percent lean grass-fed ground turkey
2 cans pinto beans, rinsed and drained
1 can cannellini beans, rinsed and drained
2 c. chopped kale, frozen or fresh
1 large or 1½ c. green pepper, chopped
1 c. chopped onion
2 c. pumpkin puree, fresh or canned
2 cloves garlic, minced
½ tsp. + 2½ tsp. cumin
½ + 1 tsp. chili powder
½ + 1½ tsp. salt
¼ tsp. cinnamon
¼ tsp. cayenne pepper
1 tbsp. Worcestershire sauce
2 c. water
1 package thin spaghetti noodles
5 tbsp. low fat grass-fed sour cream
⅓ c. shredded sharp cheddar cheese

Directions:

Prepare 1 package of noodles according to directions.

In a large pot over medium heat combine the ground turkey, green pepper, onion, garlic, ½ tsp. chili powder, ½ tsp. cumin, and ½ tsp. salt. Cook until turkey meat is browned. Add the beans, pumpkin, water, the rest of the seasonings (including Worcestershire sauce) and kale. Reduce heat, cooking over a slow boil for about 10 minutes.

Serve chili on top of ⅕ of noodles, topped with 1 tbsp. sour cream, and 2 tbsp. cheddar cheese.

Nutrition per serving is approximately:

510 calories, 11 g fat, 70 g carbohydrate, 21 g fiber, 38 g protein, 580 percent vitamin A, 25 percent B12, 20 percent B6, 100 percent vitamin C, 0 percent vitamin D, 22 percent copper, 57 percent folate, 4 percent vitamin E, 50 percent iron, 25 percent calcium, 49 percent manganese, 25 percent magnesium, 7 percent Niacin, 5 percent pantothenic acid, 25 percent phosphorus, 10 percent riboflavin, 23 percent selenium, 21 percent thiamin, 35 percent zinc

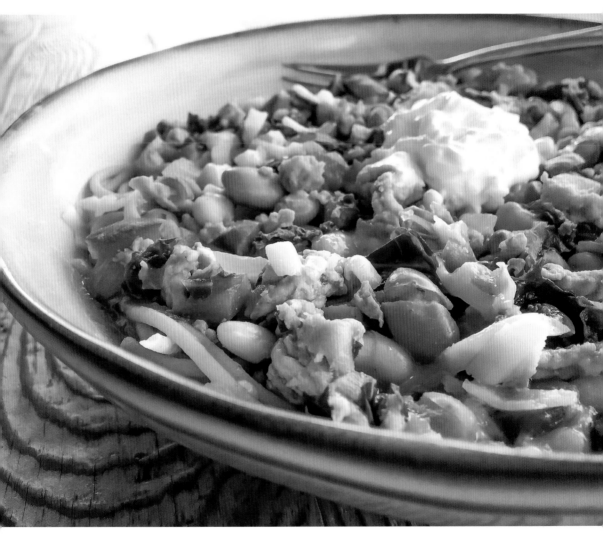

Pumpkin Chili

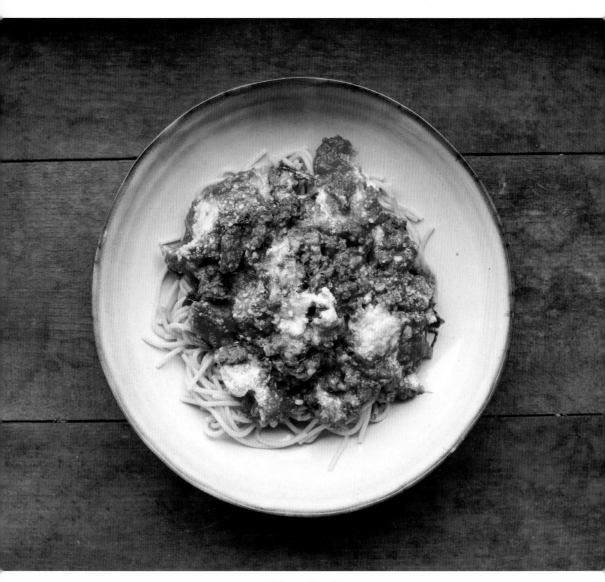

Bison Pasta

Finish Line Fueling

Bison Pasta

SERVES 5
TOTAL TIME: 30 MINUTES

GLUTEN-FREE, B12, IRON, OMEGA-3

This meal will quickly become a family favorite. Grass-fed bison is a lean protein source that carries valuable nutrients every runner requires to perform at a high level, including iron, B12, zinc, and omega-3 fatty acids. This bison pasta includes rich flavor with a touch of ricotta and Parmesan cheese. Go heavy on the noodles relative to toppings if using this meal as part of a carbohydrate countdown meal.

Ingredients:

16 ounces 90 percent lean grass-fed bison, ground
⅓ c. chopped onion
4 c. baby arugula
½ tsp. minced garlic
1 tsp. oregano
¼ tsp. salt
⅔ c. ricotta cheese, whole milk
¼ c. grated Parmesan cheese
2¼ c. marinara sauce
cooked gluten-free pasta noodles
1 tbsp. extra virgin olive oil
½ tsp. garlic powder

Directions:

Cook the pasta according to directions. While the pasta is cooking, brown the bison in a large skillet over medium heat with salt, garlic, and onion. Add arugula and oregano, cooking until arugula is wilted. Toss the bison meat with 1 c. of marinara sauce. Spread bison mixture evenly over the large skillet and drop tablespoon size dollops of ricotta cheese on drop of the bison mixture. Without disrupting the dollops of ricotta, evenly dollop and gently spread the remaining marinara sauce over the bison mixture. Sprinkle the ricotta cheese the Parmesan cheese evenly over the mixture and cover with a lid. Cook over medium-low heat for about 3 to 5 minutes, until the ricotta shows signs of beginning to melt.

Toss the cooked pasta with olive oil and ½ tsp. garlic powder. Using a large spatula top 1½ c. pasta noodles with bison mixture. Serve immediately.

Nutrition per serving is approximately:

563 calories, 16 g fat, 721 mg sodium, 841 mg potassium, 65 g carb, 5 g fiber, 34 g protein, 20 percent vitamin A, 36 percent B12, 23 percent B6, 21 percent vitamin C, 0 percent vitamin D, 10 percent vitamin E, 20 percent calcium, 22 percent copper, 38 percent folate, 34 percent iron, 22 percent magnesium, 41 percent manganese, 29 percent niacin, 7 percent pantothenic acid, 41 percent phosphorus, 23 percent riboflavin, 91 percent selenium, 31 percent thiamin, 31 percent zinc, 110 mg omega-3

Chicken, Zucchini, and Wild Rice

SERVES 4
TOTAL TIME: 45 MINUTES

VEGETARIAN, VEGAN, GLUTEN-FREE, PRE-RUN, RECOVERY

A basic rice dish can be big and beautiful with nutrient-rich vegetables. Any assortment of vegetables will do—be creative. Zucchini, onion, squash, corn, bell pepper, mushroom, and green leafy vegetables are just a few examples of greens that pair well with rice.

Ingredients:

8-oz. package wild rice
16 ounces chicken breast
   (about 2 breasts)
1 c. chopped onion
1 tbsp. olive oil
4 c. zucchini (about 4 medium
   zucchini)
1½ c. frozen roasted corn
1 tsp. sea salt
¼ tsp. black pepper
½ tsp. garlic powder
2 tsp. minced fresh sage
¾ tsp. ground ginger
¼ tsp. ground allspice
additional salt to taste (optional)

Directions:

Boil the wild rice as directed according to the package. In a large skillet over medium heat add the olive oil and onion. Allow the onion to sauté for about a minute. Add the chicken to the onion sauté and cook until it is browned and nearly cooked through.

Add the zucchini, corn, spices, salt, and black pepper. Cover and let the mixture cook for about another 10 minutes until the zucchini is soft. Finally, stir in the cooked wild rice.

Remove from heat, cover, and let it rest for a few minutes before serving.

Tip: make this meal meat free by substituting 1 to 1½ c. of white beans or 2 c. tofu for the chicken.

Nutrition per serving is approximately:

506 calories, 11 g fat, 607 mg sodium, 1,128 mg potassium, 70 g carb, 9 g fiber, 37 g protein, 46 percent vitamin A, 8 percent B12, 45 percent B6, 28 percent vitamin C, 0 percent vitamin D, 7 percent vitamin E, 6 percent calcium, 25 percent copper, 30 percent folate, 18 percent iron, 40 percent magnesium, 58 percent manganese, 86 percent niacin, 17 percent pantothenic acid, 53 percent phosphorus, 25 percent riboflavin, 33 percent selenium, 22 percent thiamin, 30 percent zinc

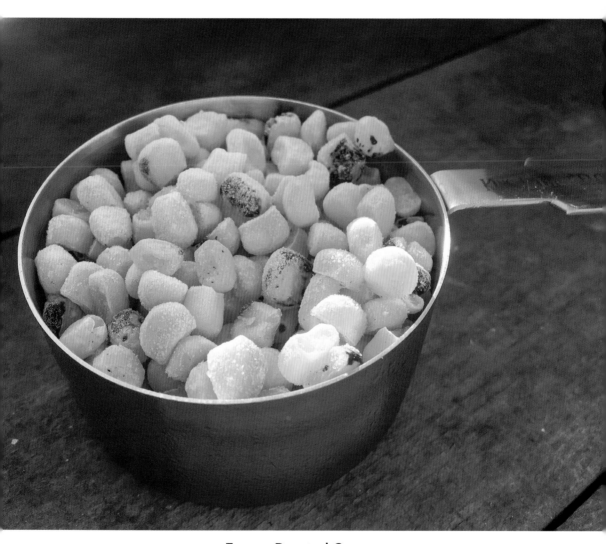

Frozen Roasted Corn

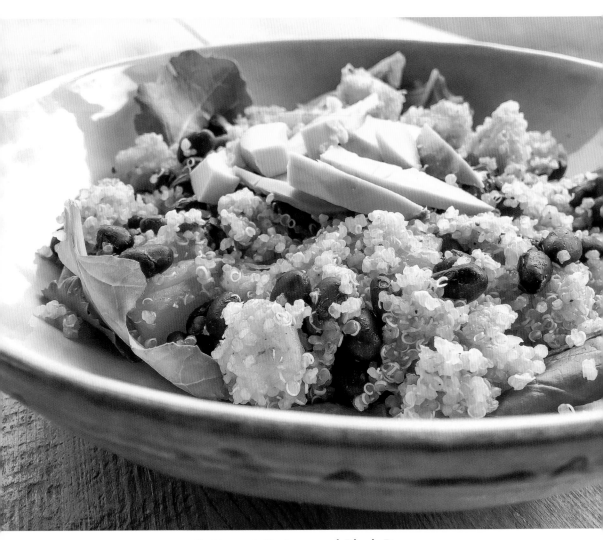

Butternut Quinoa and Black Beans

Finish Line Fueling

Butternut Quinoa and Black Beans

SERVES 2
TOTAL TIME: 10 MINUTES

VEGAN, VEGETARIAN, GLUTEN-FREE, QUICK-TO-FIX, IRON, MAGNESIUM

In a perfect world there would be enough time in the day to work in all of the necessary food prep and cooking to make a perfect meal at all times. In keeping things practical, consider the freezer an excellent resource for quality ingredients. Skip the fast food or packaged frozen dinner. This quick-to-fix, nutrient-dense option will support demanding training and a fatiguing schedule. Consider pairing this meal with a cup of milk to boost the vitamin D, B12, calcium, and zinc content of the meal.

Ingredients:

2 c. frozen quinoa, cooked
2 c. frozen butternut squash, cooked
1 c. black beans, canned and rinsed
2 tsp. olive oil
2 tsp. dried sage
½ tsp. salt to taste
½ ripe avocado, diced
2 c. kale

Directions:

Combine salt, oil, and squash in a medium saucepan over medium-low heat. Cover with a lid and let the squash cook until completely thawed. Toss in the sage and quinoa. Top the mixture with black beans and cover with the lid. Once the dish is completely warmed top ½ of the quinoa mixture on a bed of 1 c. baby kale. Place ½ of the diced avocado on top and serve.

Nutrition per serving is approximately:

504 calories, 15 g fat, 568 mg sodium, 1,261 mg potassium, 80 g carb, 21 g fiber, 19 g protein, 339 percent vitamin A, 0 percent B12, 19 percent B6, 97 percent vitamin C, 0 percent vitamin D, 9 percent vitamin E, 17 percent calcium, 46 percent copper, 70 percent folate, 31 percent iron, 68 percent magnesium, 47 percent manganese, 19 percent niacin, 17 percent pantothenic acid, 44 percent phosphorus, 57 percent riboflavin, 3 percent selenium, 38 percent thiamin, 20 percent zinc

Gnocchi Primavera

SERVES 4
TOTAL TIME: 10 MINUTES

VEGETARIAN, PRE-RACE, RECOVERY

I first discovered a similar recipe years ago in *Eating Well* magazine. It has become a favorite pre-race meal when I host my family for the Indianapolis Monumental Marathon. It's a consistent home run in terms of flavor and great marathon performances.

For a carbohydrate stocking meal, consider pairing this meal with a slice of sourdough bread. For a lower fat content, carbohydrate focused meal, limit butter to very a thin spread on the bread and reach for an extra slice to maximize carbohydrate intake. The gnocchi can easily be substituted with any form of pasta, including gluten-free, or brown rice.

Ingredients:

1 lb. potato gnocchi
2 tbsp. unsalted butter
3 cloves garlic, minced
2 large zucchini, shaved into thin
    slices with a vegetable peeler
1 pint grape tomatoes, halved
¼ tsp. nutmeg
¼ to ½ tsp. salt, to taste
¼ c. shredded or grated Parmesan
    cheese
¼ c. chopped parsley
few dashes of pepper (optional)

Directions:

Bring a medium pot of water to a boil. Boil gnocchi following directions on package.

While the water comes to a boil, melt butter in a large skillet over medium heat. Add garlic and sauté 1 to 2 minutes. Then add zucchini, tomatoes, nutmeg, salt, and black pepper. Cook until tomatoes are just starting to break down. Combine vegetable sauté with cooked gnocchi. Stir in parsley. Sprinkle with Parmesan.

Nutrition is approximately:

330 calories, 9 g fat, 49 g carbohydrate, 5 g fiber, 11 g protein, 562 mg sodium, 292 mg potassium, 44 percent vitamin A, 2 percent B12, 5 percent B6, 0 percent vitamin D, 70 percent vitamin C, 2 percent vitamin E, 11 percent calcium, 5 percent copper, 6 percent folate, 6 percent iron, 7 percent magnesium, 11 percent manganese, 3 percent niacin, 2 percent pantothenic acid, 10 percent phosphorus, 4 percent riboflavin, 3 percent selenium, 3 percent thiamin, 3 percent zinc

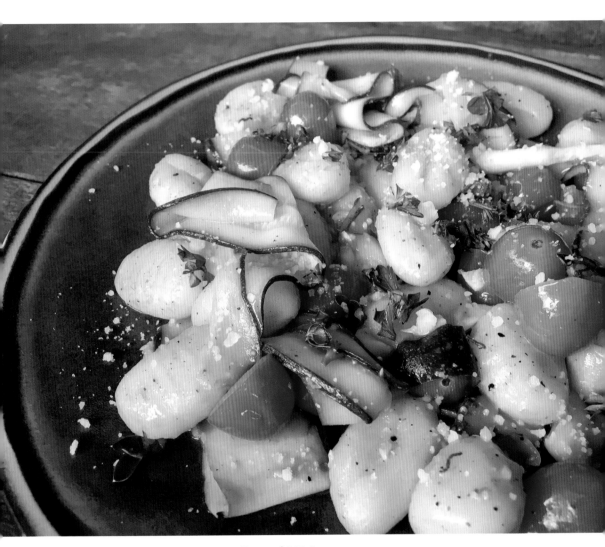

Gnocchi Primavera

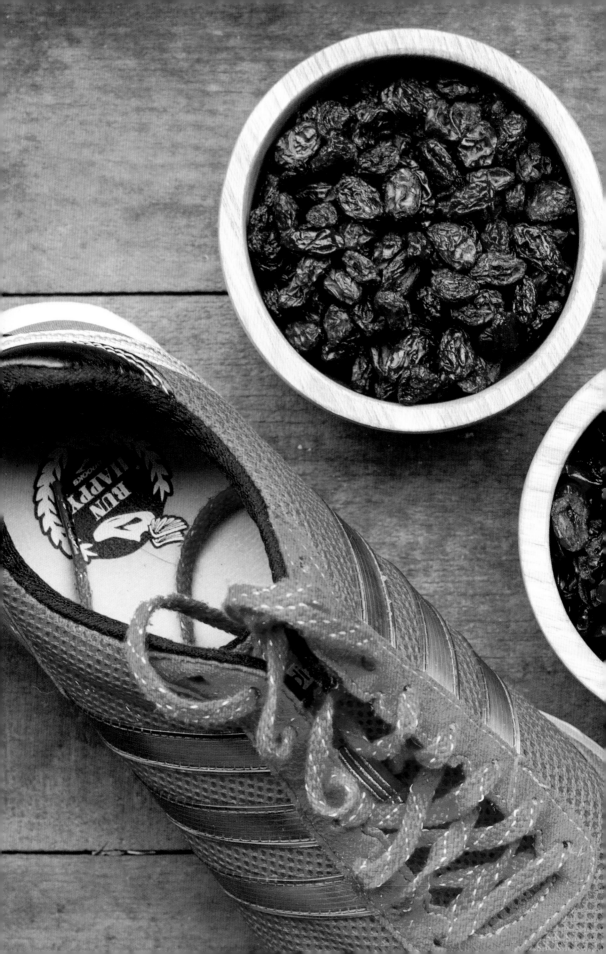

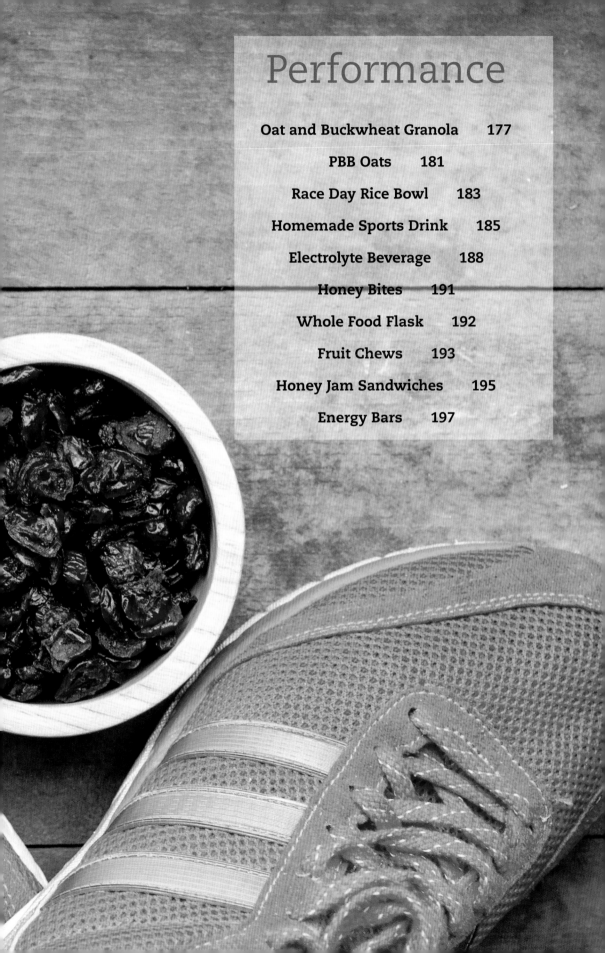

Performance

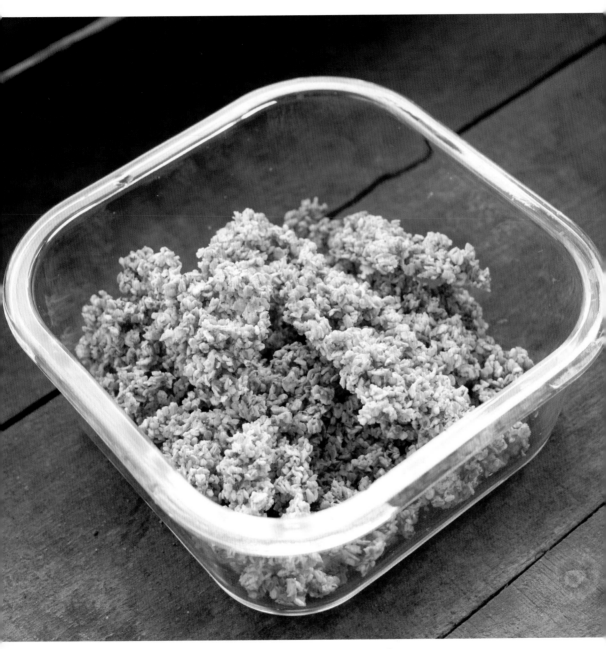

Oat and Buckwheat Granola

Oat and Buckwheat Granola

SERVES 8
TOTAL TIME: 20 MINUTES

VEGETARIAN, VEGAN, GLUTEN-FREE, QUICK-TO-FIX, PRE-RACE, RECOVERY

A goal shared by every runner is to develop a pre-race routine with familiar foods. Destination racing can throw a wrench in routine due to race weekend travel circumstances. Packing everyday food choices while traveling will support maintaining routine, put nerves at ease, and leave you feeling race ready.

Oat and buckwheat granola is an easy option to test at home as part of everyday training. If the recipe leaves you feeling well fueled and easy to digest, it will make a great option to take on the road and incorporate as part of a pre-race fueling routine. It's fast, easy, and delicious!

Ingredients:

3 tbsp. almond butter (grind fresh almonds at the grocery store to make butter as available)
3 tbsp. pure maple syrup
½ tsp. pure vanilla extract
½ tsp. sea salt
1 c. quick cooking oats
½ c. creamy buckwheat hot cereal (or slightly ground buckwheat oats)

Directions:

Preheat oven to 275 degrees. Stir together almond butter, maple syrup, vanilla extract, and salt. Add oats and buckwheat until mixture is moist and well combined. Pour mixture onto a baking sheet and bake for about 13 to 15 minutes. Mixture should be slightly wet and just starting to brown. Remove and cool.

Nutrition is approximately:

130 calories, 4 g fat, 135 mg sodium, 62 mg potassium, 21 g carbohydrate, 3 g fiber, 3.5 g protein, 0 percent vitamin A, 0 percent B12, 2 percent B6, 0 percent vitamin C, 0 percent vitamin D, 6 percent vitamin E, 2 percent calcium, 8 percent copper, 2 percent folate, 6 percent iron, 15 percent magnesium, 28 percent manganese, 4 percent niacin, 3 percent pantothenic acid, 7 percent phosphorus, 4 percent riboflavin, 5 percent selenium, 6 percent thiamin, 9 percent zinc

Race Planning with Oat and Buckwheat Granola

Tasty Destination Race Weekend Modifications:

- Top plain Greek yogurt with fresh fruit and granola for an energizing snack instead of munching on unknown race expo samples.
- Combine granola with dried cherries and a pinch of chocolate chips to satisfy a carb-loading sweet tooth instead of reaching for candy and cookies.
- Make the granola into a satisfying porridge. Combine ½ c. granola with ½ c. water or milk and heat in a microwave for 1½ to 2 minutes or heat on the the stovetop. Top the hot porridge with your favorite toppings such as fresh banana, leftover granola for texture, and a dollop of Greek yogurt.

Pre-Race Planning:

Want to incorporate oat and buckwheat granola as part of a pre-race meal? Test the example plan below as a nice starting place to assess in training and adjust based on personal preferences.

Wake two hours before any race start, from 5K through marathon distance:

1. **Hydrate:** Start with hydration. Drink 16 to 20 swallows of water upon waking.
2. **Get Moving:** Over the course of the morning sip a warm beverage to encourage a pre-race bowel movement and minimize the risk of gastrointestinal distress.
3. **Pre-Race Meal:** 90 minutes before race start, combine ½ c. granola with ½ c. water and a pinch of salt. Heat the granola mixture in the microwave or on the stovetop to desired porridge consistency. Stir in a medium chopped or mashed banana. Add a little extra protein by topping off the porridge with 4 ounces of plain Greek yogurt. This meal offers 50 grams of carbohydrate and 11 grams of protein per hour before race start.
4. **Caffeine:** Caffeine responders will want to drink their favorite cup of caffeine about 60 to 75 minutes before the race start.
5. **Stay Hydrated:** Drink any additional water; electrolyte-only beverage, or sports drink as needed in effort to achieve light-colored urine.
6. **Final Top Off:** About 10 to 20 minutes before the race start drink about 7 to 10 ounces of fluid.

Tip: This pre-race meal offers roughly 455 calories, 7 g fat, 76 g of carbohydrate, 8 g fiber, and 17 g protein.

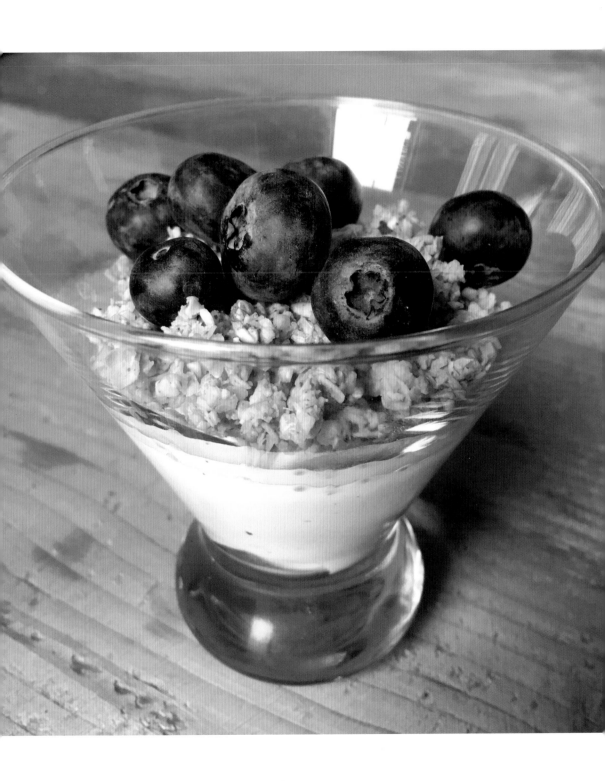

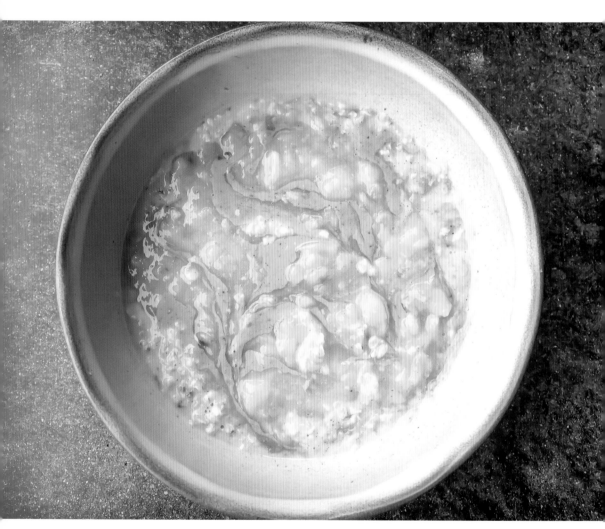

Peanut Butter Banana Oats

PBB Oats

VEGETARIAN, VEGAN, GLUTEN-FREE, PRE-RUN, RECOVERY, MAGNESIUM

There are a group of runners I have dubbed as "stick-to-your-gut" runners. These runners feel very strongly about having peanut butter, a source of good fat, as part of the pre-race meal. They feel peanut butter makes the meal feel substantial and complete. There are many ways to accomplish this goal. Peanut butter banana oats works great as a pre-race option. Pair the oats with a sports drink, kefir, or a crunchy layer of buckwheat granola to top off carbohydrate needs.

Ingredients:

½ c. quick cooking oats
6 oz. boiling water
1 large very ripe banana, mashed
1 tbsp. creamy peanut butter
1 tsp. honey
⅛ tsp. cinnamon
Pinch of salt

Directions:

Combine oats and water in a cereal bowl and cover with a plate for 3 to 5 minutes. Combine honey with the banana. Remove the plate from the oats and add the cinnamon to combine. Evenly top cinnamon oatmeal with the honey banana. Add small dollops of the peanut butter throughout the banana mixture. Run the tip of a knife through the topping to add bits of peanut butter throughout the banana mixture and serve.

Nutrition is approximately:

387 calories, 11 g fat, 67 g carbohydrates, 8 g fiber, 11 g protein, 288 mg sodium, 595 mg potassium, 2 percent vitamin A, 0 percent B12, 43 percent B6, 21 percent vitamin C, 0 percent vitamin D, 11 percent vitamin E, 4 percent calcium, 24 percent copper, 12 percent folate, 15 percent iron, 30 percent magnesium, 88 percent manganese, 16 percent niacin, 9 percent pantothenic acid, 24 percent phosphorus, 12 percent riboflavin, 19 percent selenium, 18 percent thiamin, 15 percent zinc

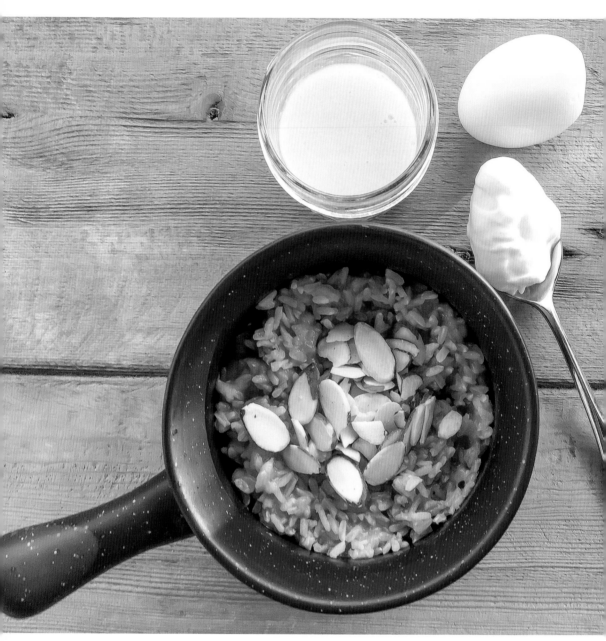

Race Day Rice Bowl

Finish Line Fueling

Race Day Rice Bowl

GLUTEN-FREE, VEGETARIAN, VEGAN, PRE-RUN, QUICK-TO-FIX, MAGNESIUM

A banana rice bowl is a great pre-race food as it offers the feeling of light and fast pre-race fueling, yet targets the carbohydrate range to support endurance performance. It works well for the runner with a nervous appetite that struggles to eat before a race by reducing the sense of volume with a mashed banana, moist texture meal. Consider serving the rice bowl with 1 hard-boiled egg, 2 to 3 tbsp. plain yogurt, or few ounces of soymilk to boost the protein content as desired. Pair the meal with a sports drink to support carbohydrate needs.

Ingredients:

1 c. long-grain brown rice, cooked
1 medium banana, mashed
2 tbsp. sliced almonds
⅛ tsp. salt
⅛ tsp. cinnamon

Directions:

Combine mashed banana, cinnamon, and salt. Add the rice to the banana mixture and top with sliced almonds. Serve warm or cold.

Race Tip: If facing warmer conditions, consider adding a touch more salt to the dish or pair the meal with an electrolyte-only beverage.

Nutrition is approximately:

364 calories, 6 g fat, 73 g carbohydrate, 7.5 fiber, 8 g protein, 276 mg sodium, 561 mg potassium, 2 percent vitamin A, 0 percent B12, 48 percent B6, 18 percent vitamin C, 0 percent vitamin D, 4 percent vitamin E, 5 percent calcium, 16 percent copper, 8 percent folate, 7 percent iron, 30 percent magnesium, 97 percent manganese, 18 percent niacin, 9 percent pantothenic acid, 18 percent phosphorus, 10 percent riboflavin, 29 percent selenium, 16 percent thiamin, 10 percent zinc

Natural Fuel

With everyday effort to limit intake of corn syrup, food dyes, and other questionable ingredients, it may feel disloyal to incorporate the undesirable ingredients when demanding the utmost from the body. But don't fear—there are many good products on the market that avoid such ingredients. Investigate sources that meet ingredient, palatability, and performance-driven goals.

There are home prepared natural options for those who would like to reduce the use of commercial sports products in training and racing. Any form of fuel, be it a homemade source or commercial, should be tested in training. Tolerance, effectiveness, preferences, and gut training necessitates proper follow through.

Keep in mind a blend of natural and commercial fuel can fit into both a training plan and a healthy diet. Alternate fuel sources between natural and commercial from one workout to the next based on practicality of fueling and resources.

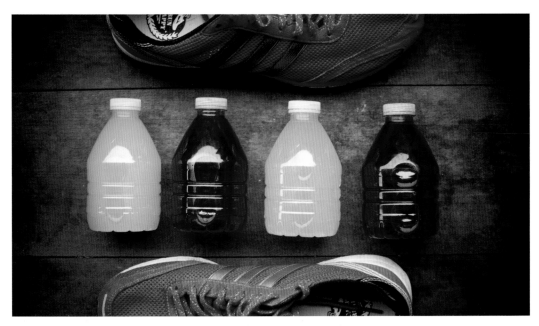

Homemade Sports Drink

Homemade Sports Drink

SERVES 4
TOTAL TIME: 5 MINUTES

VEGETARIAN, VEGAN, PRE-RUN, POST-RUN, ON-THE-RUN,
GLUTEN-FREE, QUICK-TO-FIX, HYDRATING

Purchase a 32-ounce water bottle for an easy transition to homemade sports drink. It is fast, easy, and fuels great training. The content of salt in the sports drink should be largely based on conditions. A high sweat loss workout will benefit from the higher range of sodium. A low sweat loss workout, or as an everyday drinking beverage, would benefit from the lower end of added salt. Add an optional small pinch of calcium/magnesium powder for a boost of electrolyte minerals. Consider using the brand Real Salt in sports drink for trace minerals.

Note: Sports drinks recipes are based on use of real salt. Adjust sodium based on sodium source.

Lemon-Lime Sports Drink

Ingredients:

2 ounces lemon juice
1 ounce lime juice
¼ tsp. salt (or more if needed)
3½ tbsp. pure maple syrup (or 3 tbsp. honey)
28 to 29 ounces cold water

Directions:

Combine lemon juice, lime juice, salt, and pure maple syrup in a 32-ounce water bottle. Add enough water to fill bottle to the 32-ounce line. Shake vigorously until the maple syrup has completely dissolved into the beverage. Drink immediately or chill and serve.

Nutrition per serving is approximately:

50 calories, 0 g of fat, 134 mg sodium, 55 mg potassium, 0 g protein, 13 g carbohydrate, 0 g of fiber, 134 mg sodium, 55 mg potassium, 0 g protein, 0 percent vitamin A, 0 percent B12, 0 percent B6, 12 percent vitamin C, 0 percent vitamin D, 0 percent vitamin E, 1.5 percent calcium, 1 percent copper, 1 percent folate, 1 percent iron, 1 percent magnesium, 29 percent manganese, 0 percent niacin, 0 percent phosphorus, 0 percent riboflavin, 0 percent selenium, 0 percent thiamin, 5 percent zinc

---

Coconut water can serve as a natural sports drink.
1 c. coconut water contains
45 calories, 25 mg sodium, 470 mg potassium, 11 g carbohydrate 100 percent vitamin C,
4 percent calcium, 4 percent magnesium 2 percent phosphorus

Cherry Sports Drink

Ingredients:

2½ ounces tart cherry juice
1 ounce lemon juice
¼ tsp. salt (or more if needed)
2½ tbsp. honey (or 3 tbsp. maple syrup)
27 to 28 ounces cold water

Directions:

Combine tart cherry and lemon juice, salt, and honey in a 32-ounce water bottle. Add enough water to fill bottle to the 32-ounce line. Shake vigorously until the honey has completely dissolved into the beverage. Chill and serve.

Nutrition per serving is approximately:

55 calories, 0 g of fat, 0 g protein, 14 g carbohydrate, 0 g of fiber, 135 mg sodium, 50 mg potassium, 0 g protein, 0 percent vitamin A 0 percent B12, 0 percent B6, 0 percent vitamin C, 0 percent vitamin D, 0 percent vitamin E, 1 percent calcium, 1 percent copper, 1 percent folate, 1 percent iron, 1 percent magnesium, 24 percent manganese, 0 percent niacin, 0 percent phosphorus, 0 percent riboflavin, 0 percent selenium, 0 percent thiamin, 4 percent zinc

Grape Sports Drink

Ingredients:

4 ounces grape juice
¼ tsp. salt (or more if needed)
2½ tbsp. maple syrup (or 2 tbsp. honey)
28 to 29 ounces cold water

Directions:

Combine grape juice, salt, and maple syrup in a 32-ounce water bottle. Add enough water to fill bottle to the 32-ounce line. Shake vigorously until the honey has completely dissolved into the beverage. Chill and serve.

Nutrition per serving is approximately:

52 calories, 0 g of fat, 0 g protein, 13 g carbohydrate, 0 g of fiber, 135 mg sodium, 67 mg potassium, 0 g protein, 0 percent vitamin A, 0 percent B12, 1 percent B6, 0 percent vitamin C, 0 percent vitamin D, 0 percent vitamin E, 1 percent calcium, 1 percent copper, 0 percent folate, 1 percent iron, 1 percent magnesium, 26 percent manganese, 0 percent niacin, 0 percent phosphorus, 1 percent riboflavin, 0 percent selenium, 1 percent thiamin, 4 percent zinc

Orange Sports Drink

Ingredients:

5 ounces orange juice
¼ tsp. salt (or more if needed)
2½ tbsp. maple syrup (or 3 tbsp. honey)
27 to 29 ounces cold water

Directions:

Combine orange juice, salt, and maple syrup in a 32-ounce water bottle. Add enough water to fill bottle to the 32-ounce line. Shake vigorously until the honey has completely dissolved into the beverage. Chill and serve.

Nutrition per serving is approximately:

50 calories, 0 g of fat, 135 mg sodium, 99 mg potassium, 12 g carbohydrate, 0 g of fiber, 0 g protein, 0 percent vitamin A, 0 percent B12, 1 percent B6, 21 percent vitamin C, 0 percent vitamin D, 0 percent vitamin E, 1 percent calcium, 1 percent copper, 2 percent folate, 1 percent iron, 2 percent magnesium, 21 percent manganese, 0 percent niacin, 0 percent phosphorus, 1 percent riboflavin, 0 percent selenium, 3 percent thiamin, 4 percent *zinc*

Believe it or not, a basic flask of honey or maple syrup with a pinch or two of salt, when paired with a homemade sports drink, can be an easy option that is comparable to commercial sports drinks and gels.

Homemade Sports Gel
2 tbsp. maple syrup + 1/16 tbsp. salt = 1 commercial sports gel
105 calories, 135 mg sodium, 82 mg potassium, 27 g carbohydrate

---

Low-Cal Lemon-Lime Electrolyte Drink

A low-calorie electrolyte drink works great for high sweat loss workouts lasting less than 60 to 90 minutes. It supports hydration and the desire to drink, for a low-calorie cost. This beverage also works fantastic in support of hydration before and after exercise.

Ingredients:

2 ounces lemon juice
1 ounce lime juice
⅛ to ¼ tsp. salt (or more if needed)
29 ounces cold water
2 ½ tsp of honey

Directions:

Combine lemon juice, lime juice, and salt in a 32-ounce water bottle. Add enough water to fill bottle to the 32-ounce line. Shake vigorously until the honey has completely dissolved into the beverage. Chill and serve.

Nutrition per serving is approximately:

4 calories, 0 g of fat, 0 g protein, 1 g carbohydrate, 0 g of fiber, 67 to 135 mg sodium, 55 mg potassium, 0 g protein, 0 percent vitamin A, 0 percent B12, 0 percent B6, 12 percent vitamin C, 0 percent vitamin D, 0 percent vitamin E, 0 percent calcium, 0 percent copper, 0.5 percent folate, 0 percent iron, 0 percent magnesium, 0 percent manganese, 0 percent niacin, 0 percent phosphorus, 0 percent riboflavin, 0 percent selenium, 0 percent thiamin, 0 percent zinc

Hourly Example Regimen

Hourly fluid goal based on sweat rate: 20 ounces per hour
Personal preference carbohydrate goal: 45 to 55 grams per hour

15 minutes—6 ounces sports drink
30 minutes—2 fruit chews with 4 ounces of water
45 minutes—6 ounces sports drink
60 minutes—2 fruit chews with 4 ounces water

Regimen Total:

Fluid—20 ounces per hour
Carbohydrates—Roughly 55 grams of carbohydrate per hour
Sodium—422 mg sodium per hour

Reminder: Avoid consuming sports drink with other fuel sources, such as solids and gels. Break up fuel sources over the course of the run. Most forms of fuel can be consumed with electrolyte-only beverages.

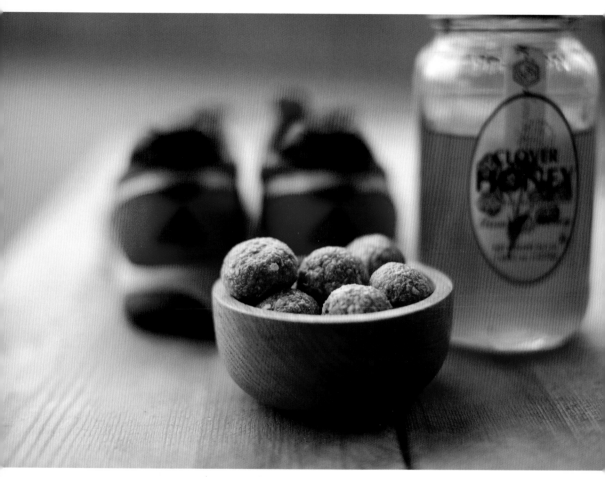

Honey Bites

Finish Line Fueling

Honey Bites

SERVES 12
TOTAL TIME: 15 MINUTES

VEGETARIAN, GLUTEN-FREE, QUICK-TO-FIX, PRE-RACE, ON-THE-RUN, RECOVERY

Honey oat bites are versatile. They work well for the track athlete between events; keep them in the refrigerator as a sweet tooth treat, or include them as part of long run efforts.

The balls can be a little soft for stowing over the course of a 3 to 4 hour run. On cold weather days they may stay firm and delicious. In warmer conditions place a small piece of parchment paper between each ball and give the ball a gentle press, making a little patty. Create a row of the desired number of honey patties between each parchment paper. Place the row of patties in a snack size sandwich bag. The snack bag can be carried, stowed behind a tree on your favorite loop, or slipped into a fueling belt.

Consider rotating the bites with other forms of fuel. A run fueled solely on honey bites may be hard to digest during harder efforts. They can be quite pleasant for a relaxed long run effort.

Ingredients:

1 c. old-fashioned gluten-free oats
¼ c. honey
1 tbsp. peanut or almond butter
¼ tsp. cinnamon
¼ tsp. salt

Directions:

Combine and stir the honey, cinnamon, salt, and peanut butter until well blended. Add oats and combine until well blended. Transfer the mixture to the food processor and mix just enough that the oats become more fine and the consistency holds together well.

Roll into 12 one-inch balls. If hands become sticky and the balls are hard to roll, wash hands and return to rolling

Nutrition per serving is approximately:

55 calories, 1 g fat, 11 g carbohydrate, 0.8 g fiber, 1.2 g protein, 51 mg sodium, 36 mg potassium, 0 percent vitamin A, 0 percent B12, 0 percent B6, 0 percent vitamin D, 0 percent vitamin C, 1 percent vitamin E, 1 percent calcium, 4 percent copper, 3 percent folate, 3 percent iron, 6 percent magnesium, 1 percent manganese, 1 percent niacin, 2 percent pantothenic acid, 0 percent phosphorus, 1 percent riboflavin, 0 percent selenium, 7 percent thiamin, 0 percent zinc

Whole Food Flask

SERVES 4
TOTAL TIME: 5 MINUTES

VEGETARIAN, VEGAN, GLUTEN-FREE, PRE-RUN, POST-RUN, ON-THE-RUN

Flavor fatigue is a common occurrence during long events fueled by thick gels and sports drink. An whole food flask offers diversity in texture that can fuel performance. Maca powder is an optional ingredient that serves as a source of vitamins, minerals, and properties that may support stress adaption, endurance, and stamina. As with all fuel, be sure to test tolerance in training.

Ingredients:

¼ c. coconut water
¼ c. pure maple syrup
¼ c. canned sweet potato puree
1 small ripe banana
¼ tsp. salt
½ tsp. maca powder

Directions:

Combine all ingredients in a small blender and blend until smooth. Pour into a flask for racing. Makes about 6 ounces, just the right size for a 7 to 8 ounces flask

Tip: Consider a single flask similar to consuming 4 gels. Be sure to pair ¼ of the flask with about 4 to 6 ounces of water or an electrolyte-only beverage, just as you would a gel, to minimize risk of GI upset. Space the maca flask contents out by rotating between the flask and other forms of fuel every 15 minutes, such as ¼ maca flask with water followed by 8 oz. sports drink 15 minutes later.

Tip: Those who are on hormone-altering medications, who are pregnant, or who have high blood pressure should consult their doctor before using maca root powder.

Nutrition for ¼ of the flask is approximately:

95 calories, 0 g fat, 24 g carbohydrate, 0.75 g fiber, 0.6 g protein, 187 mg sodium, 194 mg potassium, 110 percent vitamin A, 0 percent B12, 14 percent B6, 0 percent vitamin D, 5 percent vitamin C, 2 percent vitamin E, 2.5 percent calcium, 4 percent copper, 2 percent folate, 3 percent iron, 4 percent magnesium, 42 percent manganese, 1 percent niacin, 2 percent pantothenic acid, 1 percent phosphorus, 7 percent riboflavin, 1 percent selenium, 2 percent thiamin, 6 percent zinc

Fruit Chews

VEGETARIAN, VEGAN, GLUTEN-FREE, QUICK-TO-FIX, PRE-RACE, ON-THE-RUN

The consistency of the fruit chews may seem a bit odd while they are made, but they are a pleasant flavor and easy to consume on the run. They break apart as a moist, spongy, easy-to-swallow source of fuel. An example of fueling with chews would be a regimen of eating 2 chews with 4 to 6 ounces of water, 15 minutes later ingesting 6 to 8 ounces of sports drink, then 15 minutes later, having 2 chews and 4 to 6 ounces of water, and after another 15 minutes, 6 to 8 ounces of sports drink. Chews can be pair with electrolyte-only beverages as needed.

Ingredients:

¼ c. + 2 tbsp. banana powder
½ c. raisins
1½ tbsp. apple juice (or water)
¼ tsp. salt (or more if needed)

Directions:

Combine all ingredients in a food processor. Pulse until the mixture forms a crumbly consistency. Mold into balls. If the batter is a touch too dry, add just a pinch more of apple juice. Avoid adding too much juice. Water can be used in place of juice if needed.

Tip: Nubeleaf brand banana powder offers the best consistency for this recipe and can be purchased in bulk quantities. It's also delicious in smoothies!

Nutrition per serving is approximately:

35 calories, 0 g fat, 55 mg sodium, 101 mg potassium, 9 g carbohydrate, 0.5 g fiber, 0.4 g protein, 0 percent vitamin A, 0 percent B12, 2 percent B6, 0 percent vitamin D, 1 percent vitamin C, 0 percent vitamin E, 1 percent calcium, 2 percent copper, 0 percent folate, 1 percent iron, 1.5 percent magnesium, 2 percent manganese, 1 percent niacin, 0 percent pantothenic acid, 1 percent phosphorus, 1 percent riboflavin, 0 percent selenium, 1 percent thiamin, 0 percent zinc

Honey Sandwiches

Honey Sandwiches

SERVES 4
TOTAL TIME: 5 MINUTES

VEGETARIAN, QUICK-TO-FIX, PRE-RACE, ON-THE RUN

Over the course of a race lasting 6 or more hours, flavor fatigue can easily set in for an ultra-runner fueling on gels and sports drink. It's nice to have options besides typical gels, chomps, sports drink, and beans. A honey or jam sandwich is an alternative to test in training that offers a somewhat less-sweet texture to fueling.

A honey sandwich is basic soft bread with honey or fruit preserves. The honey soaked texture of the bread makes for a super moist, carb-rich fueling option. Consider adding a dash or two of salt to the honey-coated bread for a little extra boost of sodium if needed.

The key with taking any of type of solids is to consume them with water or an electrolyte only beverage. Eating them without sufficient fluids or with carbohydrate-rich fluids can contribute to risk of gastrointestinal upset.

Ingredients:

2 slices potato or soft bread
2 tbsp. honey

Directions:

Evenly spread the honey on one slice of bread. Sprinkle a pinch of salt on honey if needed for additional sodium. Top the other slice of bread over the honey slice and cut into fourths. One serving is one fourth of a honey sandwich.

Tip: Salted and cooked small new potatoes are another great easy-to-digest option for fueling long events.

Nutrition per serving is approximately:

80 calories, 0.5 g fat, 95 mg sodium, 5 mg potassium, 18 g carbohydrate, 0.5 g fiber, 1.5 g protein, 0 percent vitamin A, 0 percent B12, 0 percent B6, 0 percent vitamin D, 0 percent vitamin C, 0 percent vitamin E, 2 percent calcium, 0 percent copper, 3 percent folate, 3 percent iron, 0 percent magnesium, 0 percent manganese, 3 percent niacin, 0 percent pantothenic acid, 0 percent phosphorus, 3 percent riboflavin, 0 percent selenium, 5 percent thiamin, 0 percent zinc

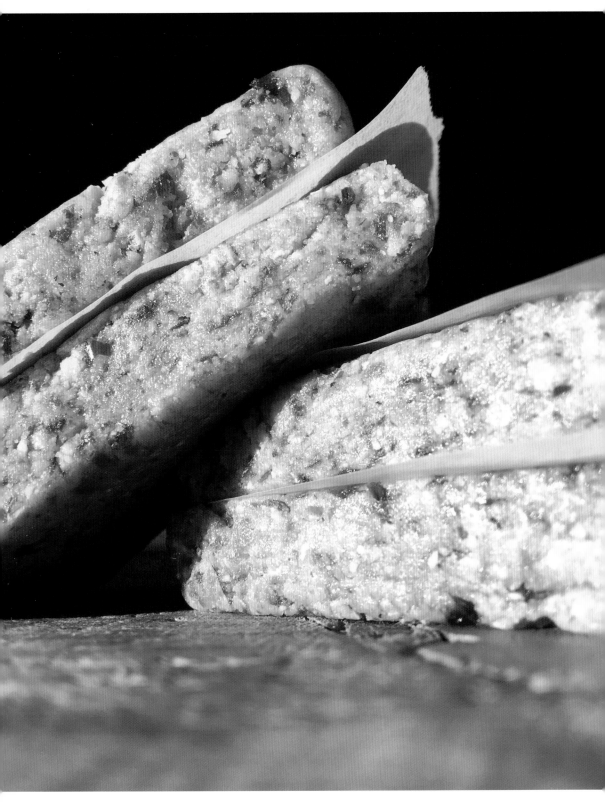

Energy Bars

Finish Line Fueling

Energy Bars

VEGETARIAN, GLUTEN-FREE, QUICK-TO-FIX, PRE-RACE, RECOVERY

Race finish refreshments tend to emphasize carbohydrates sourced from sports drink, fresh fruit, and cookies. Finding a source of post-race protein is more of a challenge. While this bar can work any time of day, it was designed as a packable post-race source of protein to help support recovery. The bar is also a touch on the salty side to support electrolyte replacement. A low mileage runner would benefit from one bar with a piece of fruit to support recovery. A higher mileage runner is likely to benefit from two bars paired with post-race fruit.

Ingredients:

4 soft Medjool dates
¼ c. pasteurized egg white powder
¼ almond flour
¼ c. quick oats
¼ tsp. salt
1 tbsp. almond butter
1 tsp. pure vanilla extract
¼ tsp. high oleic safflower oil
1 tbsp. + 1 tsp. pure maple syrup
1 packed tbsp. raisins

Directions:

In a food processor combine dates, egg white powder, almond flour, oats, and salt. Blend until the consistency looks like a slightly wet powder. Add the almond butter, vanilla extract, safflower oil, and maple syrup and blend until the mixture is completely combined and has somewhat wet consistency. Add the raisins and pulse the food processor until the raisins are blended, but small chunks of raisins remain. Remove batter by hand and gently form into a ball. If the batter seems slightly dry, mold the batter after a quick rinse and dry of your hands. The slight moisture to your hands will add just enough hydration. Mold the batter into a ½-inch thick 2 x 8-inch bar. Cut the bar into 4 even pieces. Best stored in the refrigerator.

Nutrition per bar is approximately:

212 calories, 6 g fat, 31 g carbohydrate, 3 g fiber, 10 g protein, 234 mg sodium, 292 mg potassium, 44 percent vitamin A, 2 percent B12, 5 percent B6, 0 percent vitamin D, 70 percent vitamin C, 2 percent vitamin E, 11 percent calcium, 5 percent copper, 6 percent folate, 6 percent iron, 7 percent magnesium, 11 percent manganese, 3 percent niacin, 2 percent pantothenic acid, 10 percent phosphorus, 4 percent riboflavin, 3 percent selenium, 3 percent thiamin, 3 percent zinc

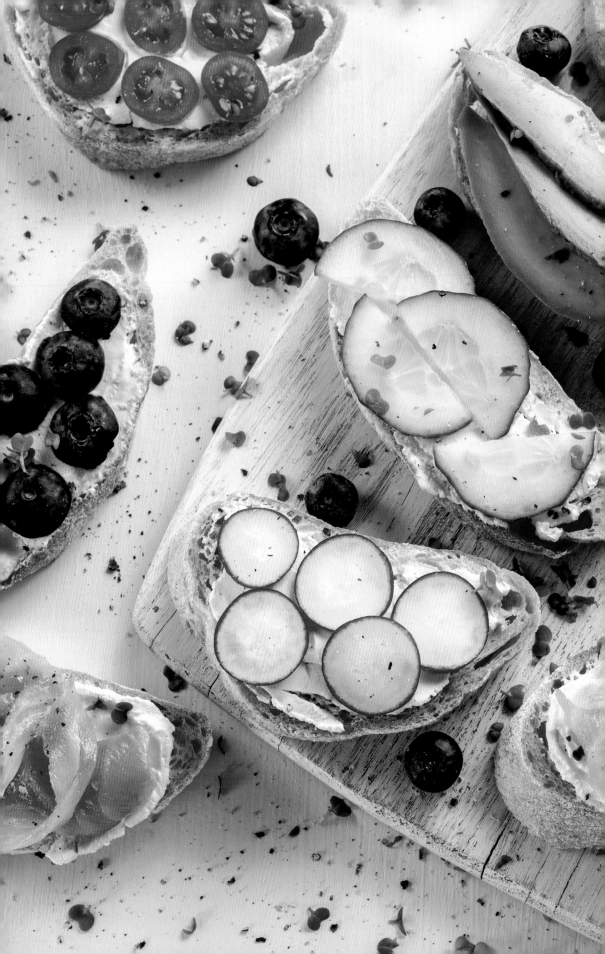

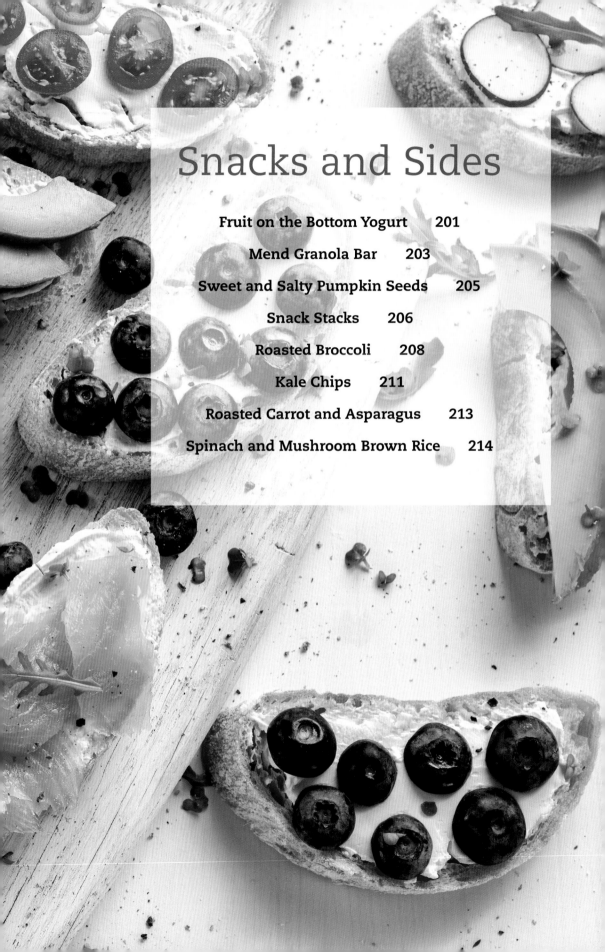

Snacks and Sides

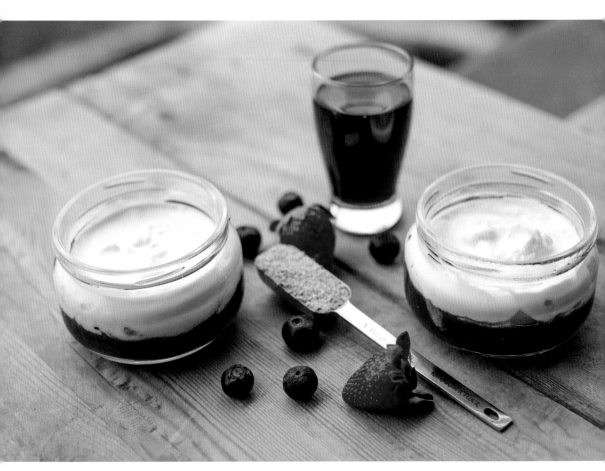

Fruit on the Bottom Yogurt

Finish Line Fueling

Fruit on the Bottom Yogurt

SERVES 2
TOTAL TIME: 15 MINUTES

VEGETARIAN, GLUTEN-FREE, QUICK-TO-FIX, B12, PROBIOTICS

Many yogurts on the shelf contain nutrient-lacking sugar sources. Making a homemade version of fruit on the bottom yogurt is fast and easy. It supports fresh, quality ingredients for everyday fueling. Use it to complement mealtime or serve as a satisfying snack. Choosing grass-fed whole milk yogurt offers as a source of health promoting conjugated linoleic acid (CLA), iodine, B12, calcium, and beneficial probiotics.

Ingredients:

Berry

1 c. blueberries
5 strawberries
2 tbsp. tart cherry juice
1 tbsp. oat bran
1⅓ plain whole milk
    Greek yogurt

Peach Plum

½ c. ripe peach
½ c. ripe plum
2 tbsp. tart cherry juice
1 tbsp. oat bran
1⅓ plain whole milk
    Greek yogurt

Directions:

In a small blender puree fruit. In a small saucepan over medium heat combine the berries, cherry juice, and oat bran. Allow the mixture to just begin to boil and remove from heat. Divide the fruit puree between two Tupperware or glass jars and let cool completely. The fruit mixture can be placed in the refrigerator to speed the process. Top each fruit puree with ⅔ c. Greek yogurt. Serve right away or seal and store for future use.

Nutrition per serving for the berry flavor is approximately:

183 calories, 6 g fat, 54 mg sodium, 294 mg potassium, 20 g carb, 3 g fiber, 14 g protein, 6 percent vitamin A, 25 percent B12, 3 percent B6, 45 percent vitamin C, 0 percent vitamin D, 4 percent vitamin E, 20 percent calcium, 3 percent copper, 3 percent folate, 2 percent iron, 6 percent magnesium, 19 percent manganese, 2 percent niacin, 15 percent pantothenic acid, 22 percent phosphorus, 27 percent riboflavin, 2 percent selenium, 6 percent thiamin, 3 percent zinc

The Munchies

Despite great fueling effort, for a hard-to-identify reason runners often pace back and forth from the fridge to the pantry trying to determine what snack will finally tide them over. Factors to rule out with hard to pacify munchies are electrolytes, fluids, and carbohydrates. Next time the munchies strike, consider some of these small snack options that can offer a big punch, and help pacify the hard-to-pin-down hankering.

- Sauerkraut or kimchi not only add probiotics, but also are a source of electrolytes. Keep a bag or jar on hand for frequent snacking.
- Kefir and chocolate milk serve as a source of hydrating electrolytes as well as carbohydrates.
- Celery is a very low calorie source of electrolytes.
- Cottage cheese can put a salty craving appetite to bed while offering as a source of protein and calcium.
- A smoothie made with coconut water or added salt can supply carbohydrates, fluids, and electrolytes.
- Be sure to pair any munchie snacking with fluids!

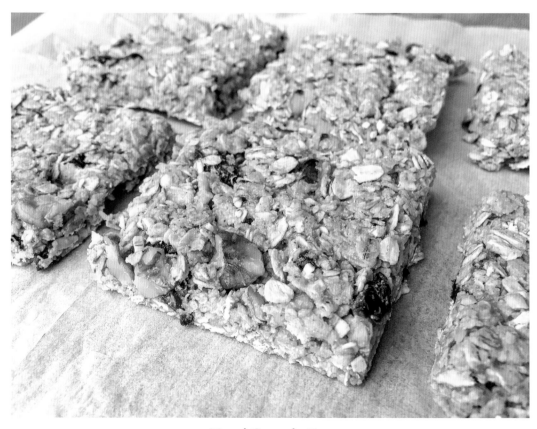

Mend Granola Bar

Mend Granola Bar

SERVES 9
TOTAL TIME: 25 MINUTES

VEGETARIAN, GLUTEN-FREE, QUICK-TO-FIX, PRE-RUN, RECOVERY

This is a go-to recipe to support endurance and health. The anti-inflammatory benefits of turmeric, ginger, tart cherries, walnuts, and complete easy-to-digest egg white amino acids fill this bar with healing flavor.

The bar is versatile in that it compares to most commercial sports performance bars marketed for endurance athletes with 248 calories, 7 grams of fat, 40 grams of carbohydrate and 10 grams of protein. Divide the recipe into 12 servings and the bar is comparable to most snack-size granola bars. Even top the bar with a little yogurt and honey for an easy dessert.

Ingredients:

1 c. gluten-free quick oats
1 c. gluten-free old-fashioned oats
⅓ c. quinoa flakes
¼ c. chopped walnuts
⅓ c. chopped dried cherries
⅔ c. unflavored egg white powder
¼ tsp. turmeric
½ tsp. ground ginger
½ tsp. cinnamon
3 tbsp. almond butter
½ c + 2 tbsp. honey
¾ tsp. salt

Directions:

Preheat the oven to 325 degrees. In a medium bowl combine oats, quinoa, walnuts, cherries, egg white powder, turmeric, ginger, and cinnamon.

In a small saucepan over medium heat combine almond butter, honey, and salt. Bring to a slow simmer. Remove and pour honey mixture on dry mixture and stir until well combined.

Press the oat mixture in a 9 x 9-inch pan lined with parchment paper. Bake for 10 minutes. Lift the bars from the pan using the parchment paper. Cool completely before cutting.

For more of a crunchy snack size granola bar texture, bake for closer to 15 minutes.

Nutrition per bar is approximately:

248 calories, 7 g fat, 264 mg sodium, 145 mg potassium, 40 g carb, 3 g fiber, 10 g protein, 4 percent vitamin A, 0 percent B12, 3 percent B6, 0 percent vitamin C, 0 percent vitamin D, 7 percent vitamin E, 4 percent calcium, 11 percent copper, 3 percent folate, 8 percent iron, 15 percent magnesium, 18 percent manganese, 2 percent niacin, 1 percent pantothenic acid, 15 percent phosphorus, 18 percent riboflavin, 8 percent selenium, 8 percent thiamin, 8 percent zinc

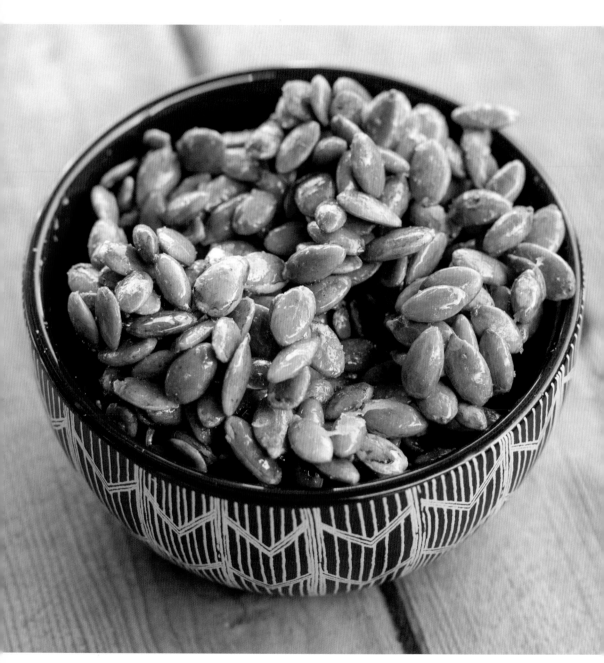

Sweet and Salty Pumpkin Seeds

Finish Line Fueling

Sweet and Salty Pumpkin Seeds

SERVES 2
TOTAL TIME: 15 MINUTES

VEGETARIAN, VEGAN, GLUTEN-FREE, QUICK-TO-FIX, MAGNESIUM

Maintaining a supply of roasted pumpkin seeds is a great go-to snack. They can add subtle sweet and salty flavor as a topping for hot porridge, salads, soups, or a smoothie bowl. Combine the seeds with dried fruit, granola, and nuts for a balanced trail mix. Pumpkin seeds are a great way for a runner to boost minerals like magnesium, copper, iron, and zinc. Keep the cupboard stocked with this mineral-rich treat.

Ingredients:

½ c. raw, shelled pumpkin seeds
1 tbsp. pure maple syrup
¼ tsp. salt

Directions:

Preheat the oven to 325 degrees. Line a baking sheet with parchment paper. In a medium bowl combine the maple syrup and salt. Toss the pumpkin seeds in the maple mixture until evenly coated. Spread the coated pumpkin seeds on the parchment paper. Bake in the oven for about 5 to 6 minutes until the pumpkin seeds slightly puff up and begin to brown. Let cool completely before storing in an airtight container.

Nutrition per serving is approximately:

206 calories, 8 g fat, 584 mg K, 11 g carb, 2 g fiber, 10 g protein, 5 percent vitamin A, 0 percent B12, 3 percent B6, 1 percent vitamin C, 0 percent vitamin D, 5 percent vitamin E, 2 percent calcium, 49 percent copper, 5 percent folate, 17 percent iron, 48 percent magnesium, 90 percent manganese, 10 percent niacin, 5 percent pantothenic acid, 57 percent phosphorus, 4 percent riboflavin, 6 percent selenium, 8 percent thiamin, 25 percent zinc

Snack Stacks

SERVES 1
TOTAL TIME: 5 MINUTES

VEGETARIAN, VEGAN, QUICK-TO-FIX

There are many versions of snack stacks that can be created. The overall concept is to stack great fueling ingredients on a slice of warm toast, lightly salted brown rice cake, or tortilla. Avocado, tomato, and nutritional yeast is one example, but there are many ingredients that can make a stack a very well balanced snack.

Ingredients:

1 slice whole grain toast, lightly salted brown rice cake, or tortilla
¼ avocado, lightly mashed
2 thick slices tomato
1 tsp. nutritional yeast
salt to taste (optional)
hard-boiled egg (optional)

Directions:

On toasted grain-rich bread place avocado, tomato, and nutritional yeast. Serve right away.

Tip: Other great stack combinations:
- Almond or peanut butter, banana, honey, and wheat germ
- Ricotta cheese, fresh peach, and honey
- Crushed pinto beans, sliced English cucumber, tzatziki
- Roasted red pepper, goat cheese, and drizzle of balsamic vinegar

Nutrition per serving with whole grain toast is approximately:

206 calories, 8 g fat, 155 mg sodium, 355 mg K, 30 g carb, 8 g fiber, 8 g protein, 7 percent vitamin A, 10 percent B12, 40 percent B6, 29 percent vitamin C, 0 percent vitamin D, 1 percent vitamin E, 11 percent calcium, 13 percent copper, 8 percent folate, 17 percent iron, 6 percent magnesium, 6 percent manganese, 21 percent niacin, 15 percent pantothenic acid, 4 percent phosphorus, 44 percent riboflavin, 3 percent selenium, 48 percent thiamin, 4 percent zinc

Roasted Vegetables

Once a routine falls into place of preparing and eating flavorful roasted vegetables, they will be a craved favorite. Toss any assortment of vegetables in healthy oil and seasoning. Place them in the oven anywhere between 400–450 degrees on a parchment paper–lined baking sheet for easy clean up. Bake for about 20 minutes, or until soft. The same basic recipe applies with any combination of vegetables in a similar ratio of about 4 cups vegetables, 1 to 2 tablespoons of healthy oil, and seasoning. The smaller a vegetable is chopped, the less time it will take to cook.

Roasted vegetables are a powerful, nutrient-dense option that can enhance any meal. I love making roasted vegetables a little on the oily side. Toss the oil-roasted vegetables on a salad, in sandwich, or with rice—no additional dressing is required. Let the wonderfully charred simple warm flavor shine through.

Green leafy vegetables are an exception in preparing vegetables for roasting. Before tossing them in oil and seasoning, but be sure to dry them with a clean cloth or paper towel after rinsing. In addition, cook them at a lower temperature, closer to 300 degrees.

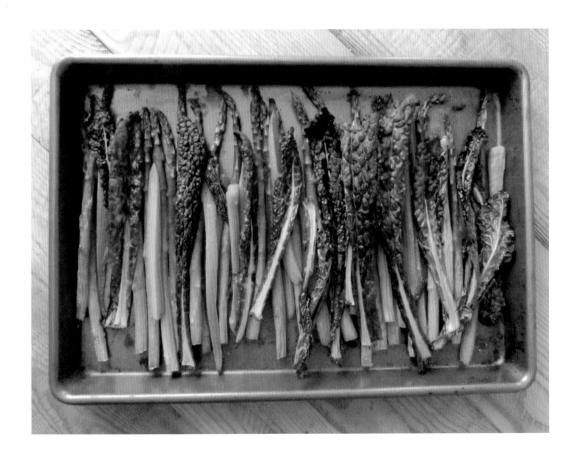

Roasted Broccoli

SERVES 4
TOTAL TIME: 25 MINUTES

VEGETARIAN, VEGAN, GLUTEN-FREE, QUICK-TO FIX, B12

Broccoli is an excellent source of the mineral chromium with a one-cup serving providing over 50 percent of daily value. Athletes have chromium loss due to high sweat loss as well as chromium loss related to a carbohydrate-rich diet. Chromium plays a very important role in support of glucose-insulin response. Making broccoli part of a regular regimen supports meeting chromium needs.

Ingredients:

4 c. fresh chopped broccoli
2 garlic cloves, minced
2 tbsp. extra virgin olive oil
¼ tsp. salt

Directions:

Preheat the oven to 425 degrees. Toss the olive oil, broccoli, garlic, and salt in a medium to large mixing bowl. Spread the broccoli evenly over a parchment paper-lined cookie sheet. Bake for 15 to 20 minutes, until the broccoli is tender and starting to brown. Serve warm or store in an airtight container in the refrigerator for easy snacking or future meal addition.

Nutrition per serving is approximately:

87 calories, 7 g fat, 292 mg K, 156 mg sodium, 5 g carbohydrate, 3 g fiber, 3 g protein, 27 percent vitamin A, 0 percent B12, 8 percent B6, 138 percent vitamin C, 0 percent vitamin D, 11 percent vitamin E, 5 percent calcium, 2 percent copper, 16 percent folate, 5 percent iron, 6 percent magnesium, 11 percent manganese, 3 percent niacin, 5 percent pantothenic acid, 6 percent phosphorus, 6 percent riboflavin, 4 percent selenium, 4 percent thiamin, 3 percent zinc

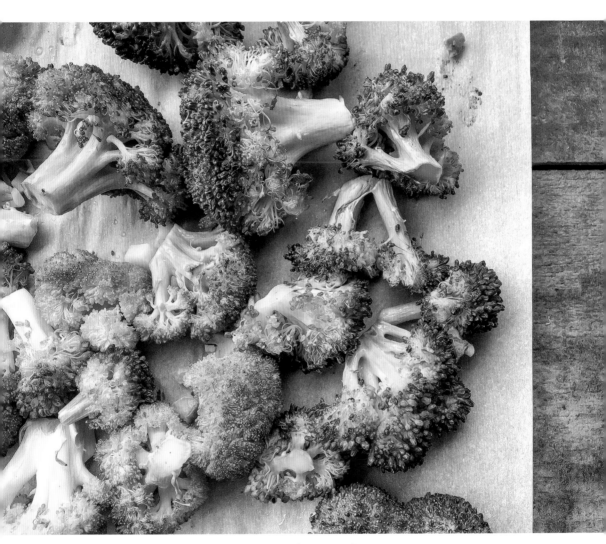

Roasted Broccoli

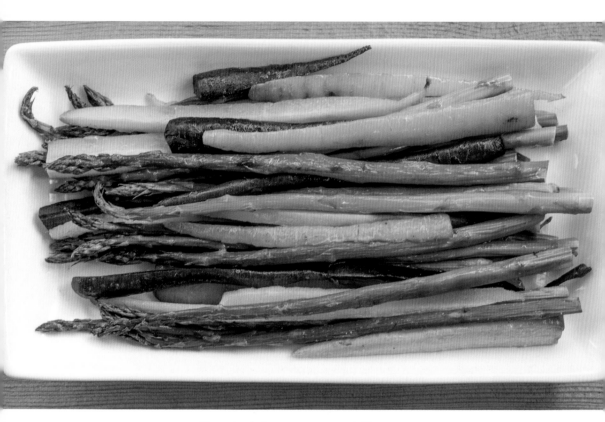

Roasted Asparagus and Carrots

Roasted Asparagus and Carrots

SERVES 6
TOTAL TIME: 40 MINUTES

VEGETARIAN, VEGAN, GLUTEN-FREE, QUICK-TO-FIX

Very little chopping and prep is involved with roasting carrots and asparagus. A quick toss in the oven allows for the rest of the meal to be prepared with little worry. Roasted vegetables are great paired with fish from the grill and rice or pasta.

Ingredients:

1 bunch of asparagus (about 20 spears)
4 to 6 medium carrots
2 to 4 garlic cloves, minced (optional)
2 tbsp. olive oil
¼ tsp. salt
few dashes of black pepper (optional)

Directions:

Preheat oven to 425 degrees. Wash the asparagus and carrots. Cut off the ends of the carrots, then chop them into fourths lengthwise. Toss vegetables with 1 tbsp. olive oil in a medium to large bowl.

On a large baking sheet lined with parchment paper, spread the other tablespoon of olive oil and top it with vegetables. Bake for about 20 to 30 minutes or until desired tenderness. Sprinkle with salt and pepper and serve.

Nutrition per serving is approximately:

70 calories, 3.5 g fat, 131 mg sodium, 340 mg potassium, 8 g carb, 3 g fiber, 2 g protein, 153 percent vitamin A, 0 percent B12, 8 percent B6, 18 percent vitamin C, 0 percent vitamin D, 9 percent vitamin E, 3 percent calcium, 6 percent copper, 20 percent folate, 4 percent iron, 4 percent magnesium, 11 percent manganese, 6 percent niacin, 3 percent pantothenic acid, 5 percent phosphorus, 6 percent riboflavin, 2 percent selenium, 7 percent thiamin, 3 percent zinc

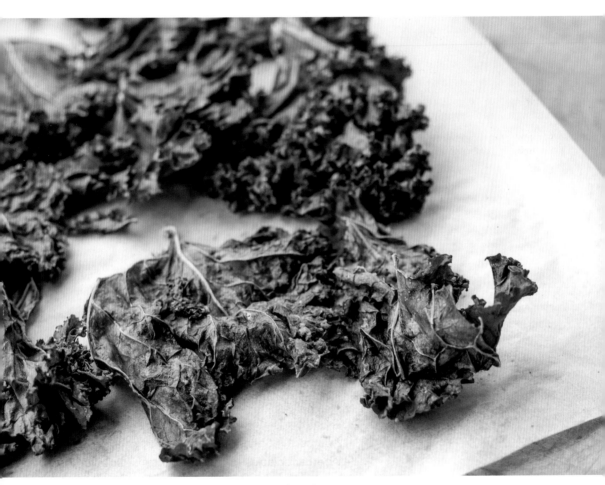

Kale Chips

Finish Line Fueling

Kale Chips

SERVES 2
TOTAL TIME: 25 MINUTES

VEGETARIAN, VEGAN, GLUTEN-FREE, QUICK-TO-FIX

Kale chips work great for an energizing salty appetite. The coating of nutritional yeast adds a delicious flavor and boost of energizing B vitamins. Pair kale chips with fruit or roasted chickpeas for nutrient dense snacking and a boost of carbohydrates. The combination of kale, nutritional yeast, and olive oil makes for very nutrient dense, low-calorie snack.

Ingredients:

4 c. kale, ribs removed and loosely chopped into large pieces
1 tsp. olive oil
1 tbsp. nutritional yeast
⅛ to ¼ tsp. salt

Directions:

Preheat the oven to 300 degrees. Line a baking sheet with parchment paper. Wash the kale and pat dry with a clean towel or paper towel. In a medium bowel toss olive oil and kale until kale is nicely coated in olive oil. Toss and coat the kale with nutritional yeast and salt. Bake until crisp for about 15 to 20 minutes. Turn kale pieces halfway through if needed.

Nutrition per serving is approximately:

103 calories, 3 g fat, 187 mg sodium, 592 mg potassium, 16 g carb, 6 g fiber, 7 g protein, 708 percent vitamin A, 20 percent B12, 88 percent B6, 178 percent vitamin C, 0 percent vitamin D, 12 percent vitamin E, 19 percent calcium, 20 percent copper, 9 percent folate, 14 percent iron, 12 percent magnesium, 54 percent manganese, 41 percent niacin, 16 percent pantothenic acid, 7 percent phosphorus, 91 percent riboflavin, 8 percent selenium, 99 percent thiamin, 73 percent zinc

Spinach and Mushroom Brown Rice

SERVES 3
TOTAL TIME: 30 MINUTES

VEGETARIAN, VEGAN, GLUTEN-FREE, PRE-RACE, RECOVERY, MAGNESIUM, VITAMIN D

This recipe is a fantastic way to boost vitamin D intake. This side dish works well paired with baked fish for a light pre-race meal.

A low fat brown rice works great for stocking glycogen stores, offering a source of vitamin D from mushrooms, and is easy to digest to keep a runner fast on their feet. Pairing rice with lean meat, dairy, nuts, seeds, or beans will offers a boost in necessary fat and protein to support a balanced meal. Consider making 2 cups of dry rice and storing leftover rice in the refrigerator or freezer for a future meal. It's a great way to make a future meal feel fast and convenient.

Ingredients:

3 c. cooked brown long-grain rice
3 c. spinach, fresh
2 packed c. sliced vitamin D mushrooms
2 portabello mushrooms, sliced into 1- to 2-inch pieces
1 Tbsp. olive oil
¼ tsp. salt
1 to 2 cloves garlic, minced
Additional salt to taste (optional)

Directions:

Cook brown rice according to directions. Combine olive oil, garlic, and salt in large skillet over medium heat. After the garlic cooks for about 1 to 2 minutes add the mushrooms and spinach. Turn off the heat once the mushrooms are soft and spinach is wilted. Add the brown rice, tossing all of the ingredients together and serve.

Nutrition per serving is approximately:

295 calories, 7 g fat, 217 mg sodium, 760 mg potassium, 52 g carb, 6 g fiber, 9 g protein, 57 percent vitamin A, 1 percent B12, 25 percent B6, 17 percent vitamin C, 133 percent vitamin D, 8 percent vitamin E, 6 percent calcium, 34 percent copper, 22 percent folate, 13 percent iron, 30 percent magnesium, 110 percent manganese, 41 percent niacin, 24 percent pantothenic acid, 31 percent phosphorus, 39 percent riboflavin, 46 percent selenium, 21 percent thiamin, 14 percent zinc

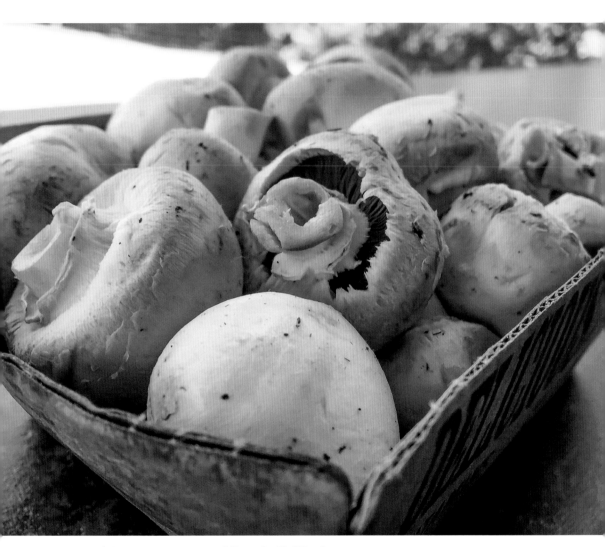

Vitamin-D Mushrooms

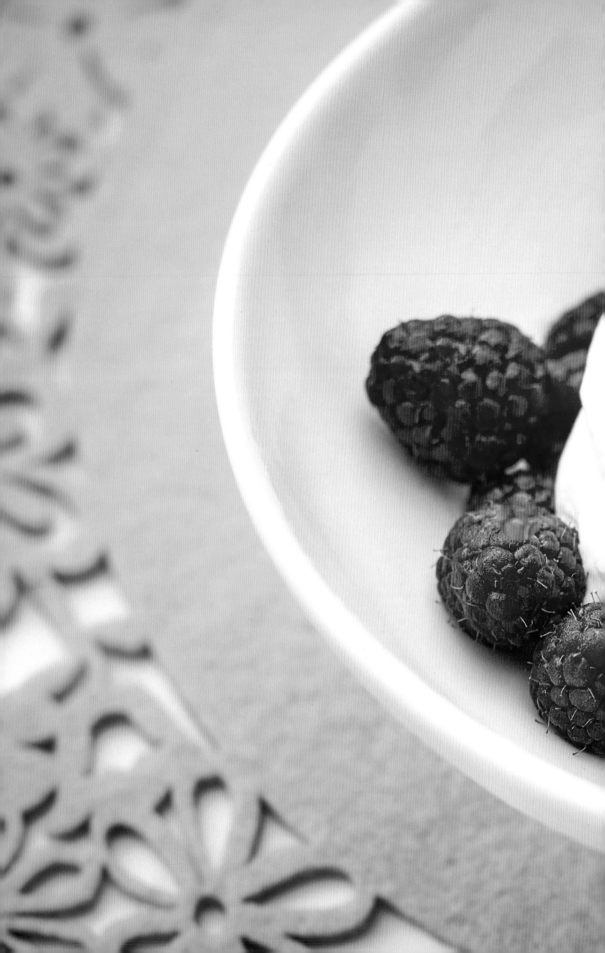

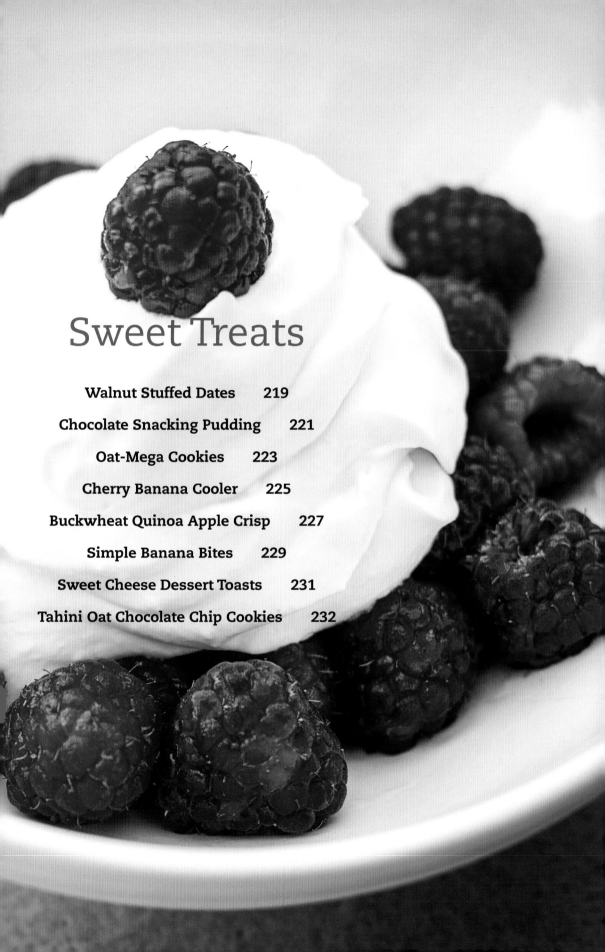

Sweet Treats

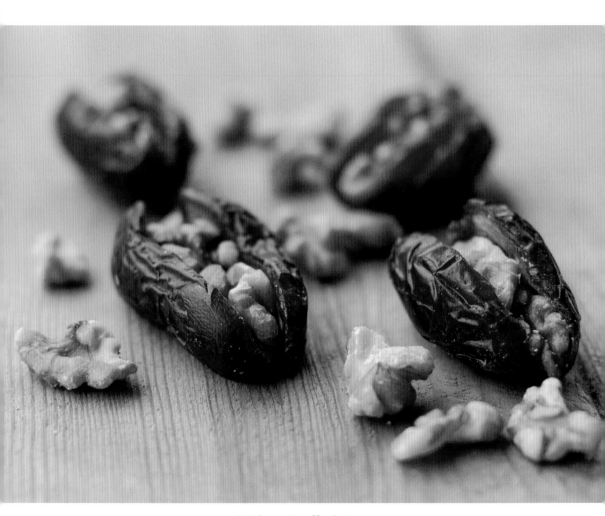

Walnut Stuffed Dates

Walnut Stuffed Dates

SERVES 1
TOTAL TIME: 5 MINUTES

VEGETARIAN, VEGAN, GLUTEN-FREE, QUICK-TO-FIX, OMEGA-3

Medjool dates stuffed with nuts are a delightful, easy alternative for candy bar cravings. The combination serves as a source of vitamins and minerals such as calcium, potassium, magnesium, B6, and more. They are also a fantastic source of fiber to support healthy bowel function and maintain healthy cholesterol levels. Stuffing the dates with walnuts adds healthy omega-3 fatty acids, copper, manganese, and many powerful phytonutrients. Sneak in a piece of your favorite dark chocolate to kill that chocolate craving.

Ingredients:

1 soft Medjool date
½ tbsp. walnuts, standard, black, or sprouted

Directions:

Cut the date halfway and remove the inner seed. Stuff the date with walnuts and gently reseal the date as much as possible. Enjoy!

Nutrition per date is approximately:

90 calories, 2 g fat, 0 sodium, 168 mg K, 19 g carbohydrate, 2 g fiber, 1 g protein, 1 percent vitamin A 0 percent B12, 4 percent B6, 0 percent vitamin C, 0 percent vitamin D, 1 percent vitamin E, 2 percent calcium, 7 percent copper, 1 percent folate, 2 percent iron, 5 percent magnesium, 12 percent manganese, 2 percent niacin, 3 percent pantothenic acid, 3 percent phosphorus, 1 percent riboflavin, 1 percent selenium, 2 percent zinc, 340 mg omega-3

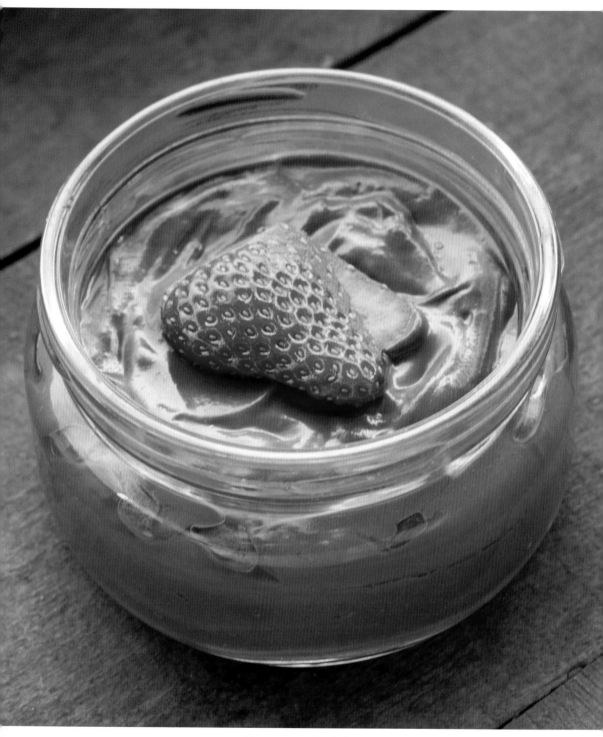

Chocolate Pudding

Finish Line Fueling

Chocolate Pudding

SERVES 1
TOTAL TIME: 5 MINUTES

VEGETARIAN, VEGAN, GLUTEN-FREE, B12, IRON, MAGNESIUM

Two common sweet tooth cravings in runners are chocolate and rich ice cream. Craving sweets may be related to a low iron status as the body yearns for a quick energy source. Runners who frequently crave chocolate often fall short in magnesium, oleic fatty acid, or both. This recipe is a fantastic source of iron, magnesium, and oleic acid—as well as many more nutrients—while satisfying a sweet chocolate craving. The fiber and fat-rich content will satisfy for hours.

A runner who struggles to maintain weight may want to enjoy this full recipe often. Those with frequent chocolate cravings may want to keep a jar of this recipe in the refrigerator as a snacking jar instead of reaching for the chocolate bowl. This low-inflammatory dessert is a fantastic fueling treat in response to a demanding training and stress load. Skip the habitual evening bowl of ice cream and whip up a batch of chocolate pudding.

Ingredients:

1 very ripe avocado
½ c. unsweetened vanilla coconut milk
2 tbsp. cocoa powder
½ tsp. vanilla extract
2 tbsp. agave syrup (maple syrup or honey)
pinch of salt (optional)

Directions:

Blend all ingredients in food processor or blender until smooth and creamy. Serve right away or serve chilled. Delicious topped with fresh berries or homemade whipping cream!

Tip: Avocado pudding is fantastic served with strawberries, banana, almond or peanut butter, cow and almond milk, plain kefir, and fresh whipped cream.

Nutrition per recipe is approximately:

516 calories, 34 g fat, 12 mg sodium, 1,333 mg potassium, 58 g carbohydrates, 21 g fiber, 9 g protein, 14 percent vitamin A, 25 percent B12, 13 percent B6, 88 percent vitamin C, 15 percent vitamin D, 0 percent vitamin E, 12 percent calcium, 70 percent copper, 31 percent folate, 14 percent iron, 38 percent magnesium, 101 percent manganese, 12 percent niacin, 28 percent pantothenic acid, 20 percent phosphorus, 11 percent riboflavin, 6 percent selenium, 5 percent thiamin, 26 percent zinc, and 14 g oleic acid

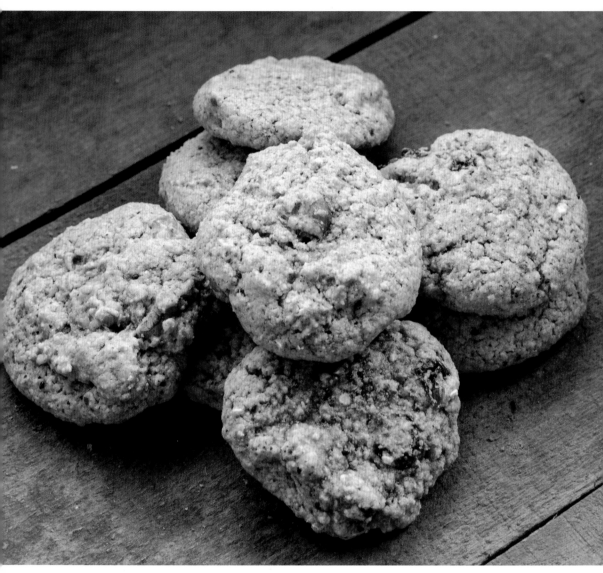

Oat-Mega Cookies

Oat-Mega Cookies

SERVES 33
TOTAL TIME: 40 MINUTES

VEGETARIAN, GLUTEN-FREE, OMEGA-3

Sugary treats should be limited, but they don't have to be lacking from the diet completely, especially if they carry quality ingredients. Each oat-mega cookie is a fantastic source of inflammation-fighting omega-3 fatty acids, using omega-3 eggs, walnuts, and chia seed sources.

Ingredients:

2 c. oat flour
1 c. quick cooking oats
½ stick butter, soft
½ c. almond meal/flour
½ c. light brown sugar
½ c. pure maple syrup
1 omega-3 large egg
1 tsp. cinnamon
1 tsp. vanilla extract
2 tbsp. ground chia seeds
1 tsp. baking soda
½ tsp. salt
½ c. raisins
½ c. loosely chopped walnuts

Directions:

Preheat the oven to 350 degrees. Combine flour, oats salt, baking soda, ground chia seeds, and cinnamon. Set to the side. Mix together butter, brown sugar, and maple syrup. Mix in the almond flour. Add vanilla and egg. Add the flour mixture to the butter mixture. When the flour is well combined add the raisins and walnuts.

Scoop the cookie dough with a heaping tablespoon and slightly roll into a ball. Place each ball onto a cookie sheet and gently press the top to slightly flatten. Bake at 350 degrees for about 5 to 7 minutes or until the bottom of the cookie just begins to brown and cookie center appears slightly doughy. Remove the cookie sheet from the oven and let cool for about 2 minutes before transferring to a cooling rack.

Nutrition per cookie is approximately:

96 calories, 4 fat, 80 mg sodium, 60 mg potassium, 16 g carb, 1.5 g fiber, 2 g protein, 4 percent vitamin A, 0.5 percent B12, 5 percent B6, 1 percent vitamin C, 0 percent vitamin D, 1 percent vitamin E, 4 percent calcium, 5 percent copper, 4 percent folate, 6 percent iron, 32 percent manganese, 6 percent magnesium, 3 percent niacin, 2 percent pantothenic acid, 4 percent phosphorus, 3 percent riboflavin, 6 percent selenium, 7 percent thiamin, 4 percent zinc, 248 mg omega-3 fatty acids.

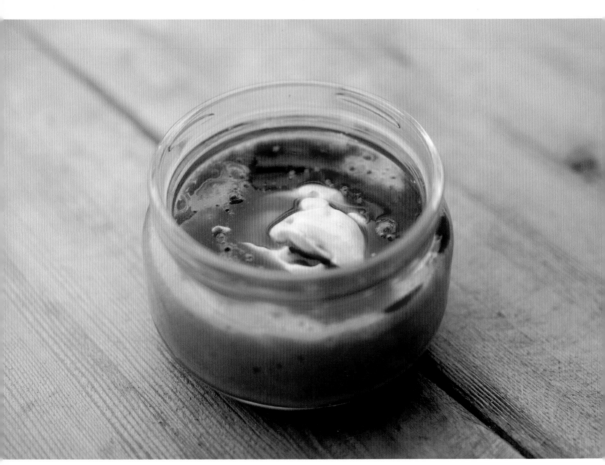

Cherry Banana Cooler

Finish Line Fueling

Cherry Banana Cooler

SERVES 2
TOTAL TIME: 25 MINUTES

VEGETARIAN, VEGAN, GLUTEN-FREE, PROBIOTICS, HYDRATING

This light and refreshing treat is great any time of day. Make a large batch in the food processor for sharing, or make a small batch. The recipe supports healthy hydration, satisfying a sweet tooth, gut balance with probiotic-rich yogurt, and inflammation fighting tart cherry juice.

Ingredients:

½ c. frozen ripe banana
2 tbsp. + 2 tbsp. tart cherry juice
3 tbsp. dairy-free yogurt

Directions:

In a small power blender, or for larger batches prepare recipe in a food processor, combine the frozen banana and tart cherry juice. Blend until smooth. Pour the banana mixture in a small bowl. Place a dollop of Greek yogurt in the center of the banana mixture. Top with a touch of tart cherry juice. Serve immediately.

Nutrition per recipe is approximately:

155 calories, 4.5 g fat, 15 mg sodium, 341 mg potassium, 26 g carb, 2 g fiber, 4 g protein, 5.9 percent vitamin A, 7 percent B12, 22 percent B6, 12 percent vitamin C, 0 percent vitamin D, 1 percent vitamin E, 5 percent calcium, 4 percent copper, 4 percent folate, 2 percent iron, 6 percent magnesium, 6 percent manganese, 2 percent niacin, 2 percent pantothenic acid, 2 percent phosphorus, 5 percent riboflavin, 1 percent selenium, 2 percent thiamin, 1 percent zinc

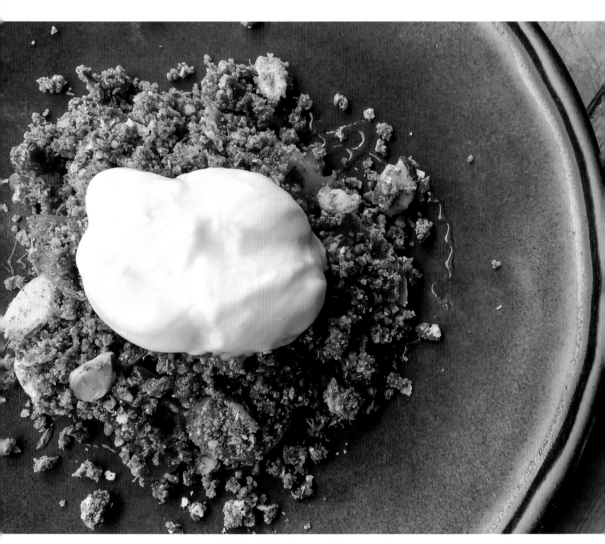

Buckwheat Quinoa Apple Crisp

Buckwheat Quinoa Apple Crisp

SERVES 5
TOTAL TIME: 30 MINUTES

VEGETARIAN, VEGAN, QUICK-TO-FIX, MAGNESIUM, PROBIOTICS

The traditional apple crisp heavy in butter, white flour, brown sugar, and vanilla ice cream can be recreated into a satisfying yet more nutritious sweet treat. Buckwheat quinoa apple crisp can work for an evening dessert or a morning brunch. Explore changing the type of fruit to peach or pear with fresh seasonal fruit.

Ingredients:

4 c. sliced apples (about 3 apples)
1 tsp. grated ginger root
1 tbsp. maple syrup + ¼ c. maple syrup
½ c. buckwheat flour
½ c. quinoa flakes
¼ + 1 tsp. cinnamon
¼ c. brown sugar
½ tsp. nutmeg
¼ c. almond slices
3 tbsp. melted coconut oil
¾ tsp. salt

Toppings:

2 tbsp. honey
5.3 oz. plain Greek or almond yogurt

Directions:

Preheat oven to 350 degrees. In a medium skillet or saucepan, combine apples, ginger, and 1 tbsp. maple syrup. Cover and allow apples to cook until soft, about 15 minutes.

In a medium bowl combine buckwheat, quinoa, cinnamon, sugar, nutmeg, the remaining ¼ cup maple syrup syrup, almonds, salt, and coconut oil. Pour cooked apple mixture in a shallow pie or baking dish. Layer the crumble mixture over the cooked apples and bake for about 15 minutes, until crumble is crisp. Top each serving with 2 tbsp. of Greek or almond yogurt and 1 tsp. honey drizzle.

Nutrition per serving with honey and Greek yogurt is approximately:

348 calories, 12 g fat, 330 mg sodium, 226 mg potassium, 60 g carb, 5 g fiber, 6 g protein, 1 percent vitamin A, 0 percent B12, 20 percent B6, 8 percent vitamin C, 0 percent vitamin D, 14 percent vitamin E, 9 percent calcium, 40 percent copper, 15 percent folate, 10 percent iron, 34 percent magnesium, 56 percent manganese, 5 percent niacin, 2 percent pantothenic acid, 33 percent phosphorus, 20 percent riboflavin, 4 percent selenium, 10 percent thiamin, 22 percent zinc

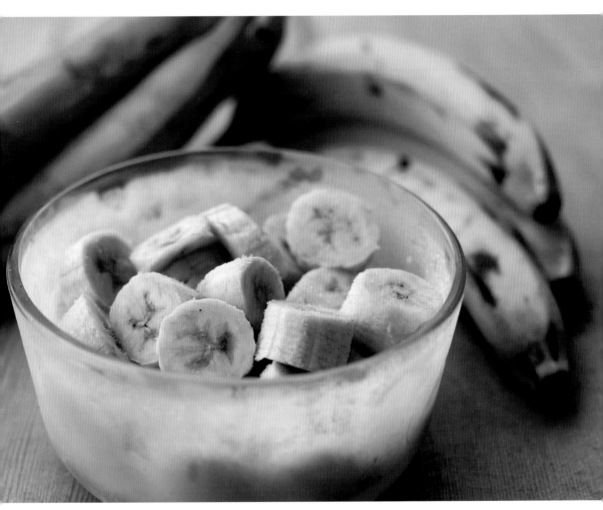

Simple Banana Bites

Finish Line Fueling

Simple Banana Bites

SERVES 4
TOTAL TIME: 4 HOURS

VEGETARIAN, VEGAN, GLUTEN-FREE, PRE-RACE, RECOVERY

It sounds too easy, right? Keep a stash of frozen sweet ripe bananas on hand at all times. This simple treat can kill a sweet tooth craving, support meeting carbohydrate goals, and offer essential runner nutrients such as magnesium and potassium. Savoring the simple frozen banana is also a great weight management strategy due to the low calorie content and slowing the time it takes to eat the banana.

Get creative with the frozen banana and blend it in the food processor to make an ice cream. Top the ice cream with extras such as a dollop of peanut butter, slivered almonds, cocoa powder, and ground flax seed.

Ingredients:

4 very ripe bananas

Directions:

Peel and slice the into 1–2-inch pieces. Place the bananas in airtight Tupperware and place them in the freezer. Once frozen snack on the frozen treat as desired. They are simple and delicious.

Nutrition per serving is approximately:

105 calories, 0 g fat, 1 mg sodium, 422 mg potassium, 27 g carb, 3 fiber, 4 g protein, 2 percent vitamin A, 0 percent B12, 22 percent B6, 17 percent vitamin C, 0 percent vitamin D, 1 percent vitamin E, 1 percent calcium, 5 percent copper, 6 percent folate, 2 percent iron, 8 percent magnesium, 16 percent manganese, 4 percent niacin, 4 percent pantothenic acid, 3 percent phosphorus, 57 percent riboflavin, 2 percent selenium, 2 percent thiamin, 1 percent zinc

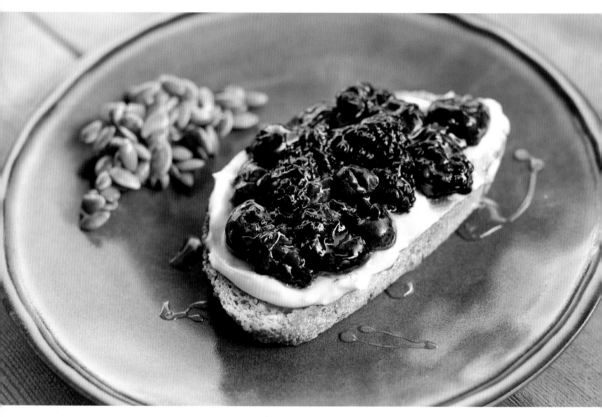

Sweet Cheese Dessert Toast

Sweet Cheese Dessert Toast

SERVES 1
TOTAL TIME: 5 MINUTES

VEGETARIAN, QUICK-TO-FIX, MAGNESIUM

Dessert toast is a sweet version of a snack stack for a no refined sugar cost. A spread of mascarpone cheese offers a cheesecake flavor topped with sweet fruit and honey. Toast makes a wonderful bed for the pleasantly sweet topping, but can be substituted with a pancake or wrap the ingredients in a warm tortilla. Dessert toast is an easy way to kill a carbohydrate craving sweet tooth without resorting to the high inflammatory candy bowl.

Ingredients:

1 tbsp. mascarpone cheese
¼ c. mashed berries
1 tsp. honey
1 slice 100 percent whole grain toast

Directions:

Peel and slice the bananas and cut them into 1–2 inch pieces. Put the bananas in airtight container and place them in the freezer. Once frozen, snack as desired!

Tip: Consider a sprinkle of wheat germ or pumpkin seeds to heighten the nutrient content of this dessert toast.

Tip: Substitute cheese for plain Greek yogurt, or blend the two together to add probiotics.

Nutrition per serving is approximately:

228 calories, 9 g fat, 170 mg sodium, 181 mg potassium, 35 g carb, 4 g fiber, 5 g protein, 5 percent vitamin A, 0 percent B12, 5 percent B6, 8 percent vitamin C, 0 percent vitamin D, 5 percent vitamin E, 16 percent calcium, 7 percent copper, 7 percent folate, 2 percent iron, 35 percent magnesium, 49 percent manganese, 9 percent niacin, 2 percent pantothenic acid, 2 percent phosphorus, 7 percent riboflavin, 26 percent selenium, 9 percent thiamin, 5 percent zinc

Tahini Oat Chocolate Chip Cookies

SERVES 24
TOTAL TIME: 45 MINUTES

VEGETARIAN, GLUTEN-FREE

Tahini is rich source of vitamins, minerals, protein, amino acids, and healthy fat. Tahini carries minerals such as magnesium, iron, and zinc, as well as healthy oleic and linoleic acids. Tahini can be added to foods in so many ways. A great option is to substitute tahini for butter in chocolate chip cookies. This chocolate chip cookie is so good no one will notice the health-motivating difference.

Ingredients:

½ c. tahini
⅔ c. brown sugar, packed
⅔ c. granulated sugar
2 large omega-3 eggs
1 tsp. vanilla
2 c. oat flour
½ tsp. baking soda
½ tsp. salt
⅔ c. 60 percent dark cacao chocolate chips
⅓ c. walnuts, chopped (optional)

Directions:

Preheat oven to 375 degrees. In a medium bowl combine the tahini, sugar, eggs, and vanilla. Then blend in oat flour, baking soda, and salt. Finally, stir in chocolate chips. Spoon the batter onto cookie sheet. Bake for about 7 to 8 minutes or until the bottom of cookie starts to brown. The middles will be slightly doughy. Remove and cool on a cookie rack.

Nutrition per cookie is approximately:

130 calories, 5 g fat, 89 mg sodium, 60 mg potassium, 22 g carb, 2 g fiber, 4 g protein, 0 percent vitamin A, 1 percent B12, 1 percent B6, 0 percent vitamin C, 1 percent vitamin D, 1 percent vitamin E, 4 percent calcium, 7 percent copper, 3 percent folate, 5 percent iron, 5 percent magnesium, 24 percent manganese, 3 percent niacin, 1 percent pantothenic acid, 9 percent phosphorus, 3 percent riboflavin, 5 percent selenium, 9 percent thiamin, 4 percent zinc

Simply Refreshing

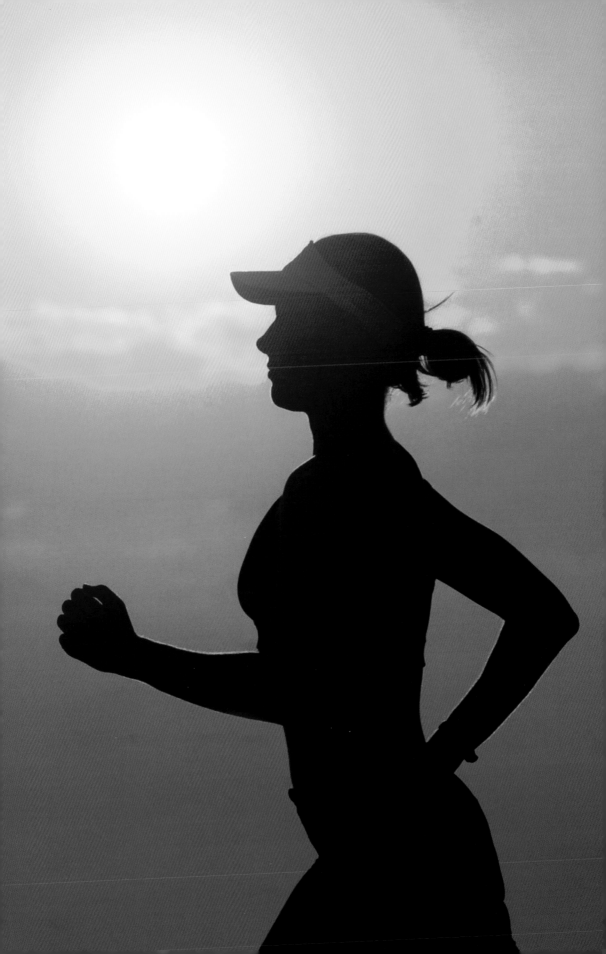

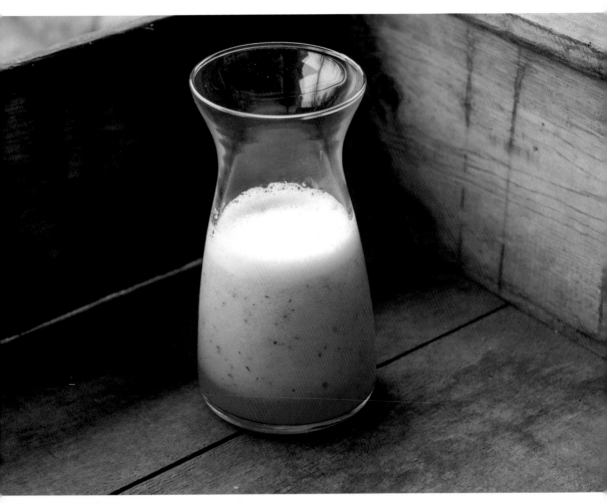

Peachy Lemon Cooler

Finish Line Fueling

Peachy Lemon Cooler

SERVES 1
TOTAL TIME: 5 MINUTES

VEGETARIAN, VEGAN, GLUTEN-FREE, QUICK-TO-FIX, HYDRATING

Here is a wonderful rehydrating treat that works great after a sweat-soaking workout or as a relaxing pick-me-up. Explore using various fruit such as peach, berries, and watermelon.

Ingredients:

½ large ripe peach
½ lemon, juiced
1 c. water,
½ c. ice
pinch of salt
2 tsp. agave nectar (optional)

Directions:

Blend all ingredients in small blender until smooth and serve immediately.

Nutrition per recipe is approximately:

40 calories, 0 g fat, 175 mg sodium, 192 mg potassium, 11 g carbohydrate, 2 g fiber, 1 g protein, 9 percent vitamin A, 0 percent B12, 2 percent B6, 32 percent vitamin C, 0 percent vitamin D, 3 percent vitamin E, 1 percent calcium, 3 percent copper, 2 percent folate, 1 percent iron, 2 percent magnesium, 2 percent manganese, 4 percent niacin, 2 percent pantothenic acid, 1 percent phosphorus, 2 percent riboflavin, 1 percent selenium, 2 percent thiamin, 1 percent zinc

Simple Green Smoothie

SERVES 1
TOTAL TIME: 5 MINUTES

VEGETARIAN, GLUTEN-FREE, QUICK-TO-FIX, HYDRATING

This smoothie base offers a nutrient-rich start or addition to the day for a low calorie punch. For the similar calorie load as a standard 8-ounce juice, this 8-ounce green smoothie serves as a source of protein, probiotics, fiber, calcium, vitamin C, potassium, copper, phenol antioxidants, iron, vitamin D, magnesium, a touch of healthy fat, and more.

Enjoy the fresh smoothie unsweetened, or add the naturally sweetened flavor and carbohydrate boost of a Medjool date. Develop the base smoothie by adding ingredients like a banana, flaxseed, berries, avocado, or protein powder.

Ingredients:

½ c. unsweetened almond milk
1 c. fresh spinach
¼ c. plain Greek yogurt
1 soft Medjool date, pit removed
2–3 pieces ice (optional)

Directions:

Combine all ingredients in blender. First add spinach, next add yogurt and dates. Begin on lower speed and increase or pulse until smooth.

Nutrition is approximately:

127 calories, 2 g fat, 135 mg sodium, 429 mg potassium, 22 g carbohydrate, 3 g fiber, 8 g protein, 62 percent vitamin A, 0 percent B12, 6 percent B6, 14 percent vitamin C, 13 percent vitamin D, 28 percent vitamin E, 34 percent calcium, 6 percent copper, 16 percent folate, 8 percent iron, 11 percent magnesium, 17 percent manganese, 3 percent niacin, 2 percent pantothenic acid, 5 percent phosphorus, 5 percent riboflavin, 1 percent selenium, 2 percent thiamin, 3 percent zinc

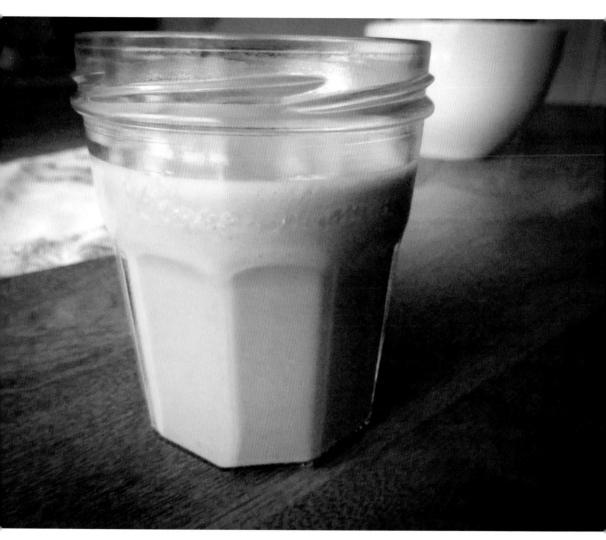

Simple Green Smoothie

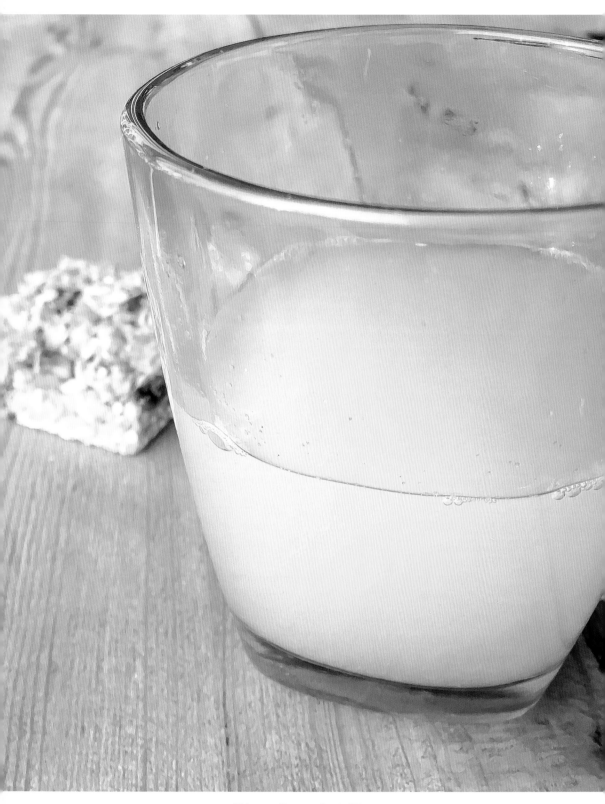

Warm Grapefruit Tea

Finish Line Fueling

Warm Grapefruit Tea

SERVES 1
TOTAL TIME: 10 MINUTES

VEGETARIAN, VEGAN, GLUTEN-FREE, QUICK-TO-FIX, HYDRATING

A benefit of tea from citrus fruit is the mega dose of vitamin C it carries. Vitamin C is a powerful antioxidant that helps in fighting off upper respiratory tract infections and aids the overall health of the immune system.

Adding honey to this tea may reduce nighttime coughing and improve sleep if signs of a seasonal cold take shape. The oils from cinnamon have been studied for their ability to inhibit growth of bacteria. Allspice also carries immune supporting phytonutrient and anti-inflammatory properties.

Ingredients:

1 grapefruit, fresh squeezed
1 cinnamon stick (or a pinch of
    ground cinnamon)
½ to ¾ c. water
1 tsp. honey
5 to 7 allspice berries (or a pinch of
    ground allspice)

Directions:

Combine the grapefruit juice, cinnamon, water, honey, and allspice in a small pot over medium to low heat. Cover and bring to a simmer for about 5 minutes. Strain into a cup and serve.

Nutrition is approximately:

90 calories, 0 g fat, 2 mg sodium, 287 mg potassium, 22 g carbohydrate, 0 g fiber, 1 g protein, 0 percent vitamin A, 0 percent B12, 2 percent B6, 90 percent vitamin C, 0 percent vitamin D, 1 percent vitamin E, 1 percent calcium, 4 percent copper, 5 percent folate, 2 percent iron, 5 percent magnesium, 2 percent manganese, 2 percent niacin, 3 percent pantothenic acid, 2 percent phosphorus, 2 percent riboflavin, 0 percent selenium, 5 percent thiamin, 1 percent zinc

Cherry Lime Spritzer

SERVES 1
TOTAL TIME: 5 MINUTES

VEGETARIAN, VEGAN, GLUTEN-FREE, QUICK-TO-FIX, HYDRATING

Quench the urge for a carbonated beverage with sparkling water mixed with a touch of fresh fruit or juices. Add a pinch of salt if electrolyte replacement is needed. Fresh English cucumber can make a wonderful beverage addition too. A runner who is trying to break a soda habit can make this drink sweeter with a touch of honey, maple syrup, agave, or stevia.

Ingredients:

8 oz. carbonated mineral water
2 oz. tart cherry juice
1 oz. lime juice
ice
pinch of salt (optional)

Directions:

Combine all ingredients and serve.

Nutrition is approximately:

37 calories, 0 g fat, 10 mg sodium, 95 mg potassium, 10 g carbohydrate, 0 g fiber, 0 g protein, 2 percent vitamin A, 0 percent B12, 0 percent B6, 10 percent vitamin C, 0 percent vitamin D, 0 percent vitamin E, 5 percent calcium, 0 percent copper, 1 percent folate, 1 percent iron, 0 percent magnesium, 0 percent manganese, 0 percent niacin, 0 percent pantothenic acid, 0 percent phosphorus, 0 percent riboflavin, 0 percent selenium, 0 percent thiamin, 0 percent zinc

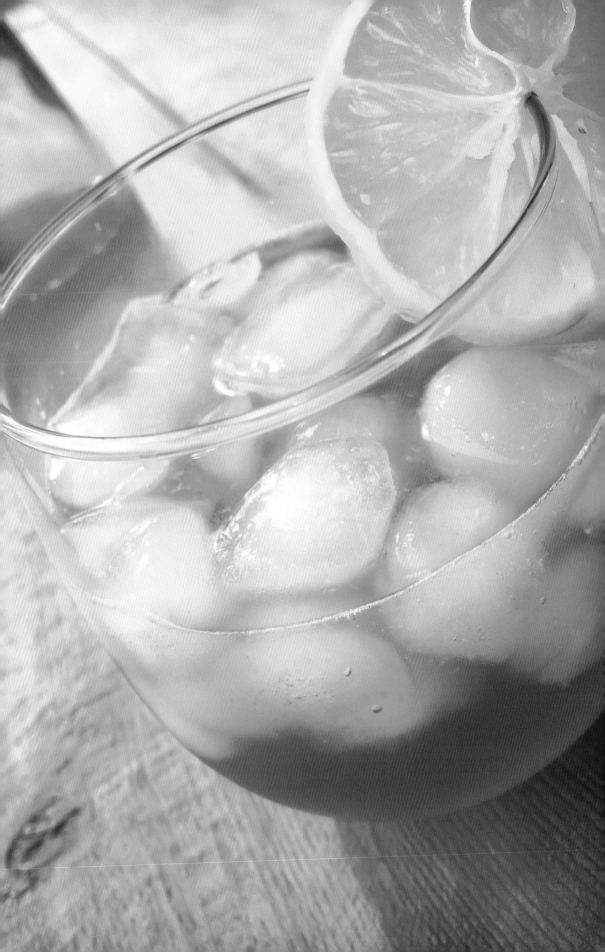